Tim,

So great to meet you. Would love to stay in touch! Please let me know if I can be of any service to you!

Neuwirth MD

P9-BZH-366

PRAISE FOR REFRAMING HEALTHCARE

Dr. Zeev Neuwirth draws upon his decades of experience—first as a primary care physician and more recently as an innovative expert in improving care delivery—to create a roadmap on how to get our broken healthcare system back on track and moving in the direction of affordable, high-quality value-based care. Turning healthcare on its head is a large undertaking, one that will require significant collaboration between informed, capable individuals. With Dr. Neuwirth's guidance, courageous consumers, employers, and industry leaders are given the tools they need to forge forward with this critical revolution.

Dave Chase

co-founder of Health Rosetta and author of *The CEO's Guide to Restoring The American Dream: How to Deliver World Class Health Care to your Employees at Half the Cost* and *The Opioid Crisis Wake-up Call*

Dr. Zeev Neuwirth writes a compelling book about how to fix what is broken in our healthcare system. He is an innovative leader focused on patient-centered care that achieves better health outcomes at lower costs. A great book from a doctor with a wonderful podcast about how to innovate and improve the health system.

Patrick Conway, MD

president and CEO of Blue Cross Blue Shield of North Carolina

Healthcare is in a state of confusion, chaos and disruption. What's needed is clarity of thought and a roadmap for effective action. Zeev delivers that in this wonderful book that explains why and how ultimately the patient as consumer is in charge.

Sami Inkinen

founder & CEO, Virta Health

cofounder & board member of Trulia

This book gives healthcare leaders a guide to do the work that we all say needs to be done. To transform our focus and cultures to truly deliver on our promises to the communities we serve. Dr. Neuwirth provides a plan that is culled from experts, experience, and insight to help you succeed amidst the turbulence.

Jeff Thompson, MD

emeritus CEO, Gundersen Health

Dr. Neuwirth is one of the brightest most authentic voices in healthcare. He is a wonderful speaker and writer and it's a real privilege to work with him and to read his thoughts. Reframing Healthcare *is a must-read for people in the healthcare world.*

Scott Becker

publisher, Beckers Healthcare

partner, Mcguirewoods

In the metrics-focused combat zone that healthcare has become, Dr. Neuwirth distinguishes himself as a patient-centered advocate dedicated to the right outcomes—reminding us all to rise about the fray. This book lays out an effective plan to address the triple aim for the future of healthcare—better care, better health, lower cost. With the Reframe Roadmap, Zeev pushes us not to just re-engineer healthcare, but to reframe it entirely.

Donald Berwick, MD, MPP

former administrator of the Centers for Medicare and Medicaid Services (CMS)
president emeritus of the Institute for Healthcare Improvement

If you think now is the time to overhaul the US healthcare system, you must read this book. Dr. Neuwirth presents us with new insights and a different approach to rethinking healthcare. This is a necessary primer for anyone interested in making the changes that will transform the healthcare system for the benefit of all Americans.

Steven S. Martin

retired CEO, Blue Cross Blue Shield of Nebraska
retired & founding CEO, Prime Therapeutics

This book is a refreshing take on rebranding, redesigning and reorganizing healthcare. It reflects a fundamentally different way of defining the problem and using a consumer mindset to create a roadmap for the future. …a must-read for senior leaders committed to truly transforming our industry.

Susan DeVore

CEO Premier, Inc.

Reframing Healthcare *offers an enticing vision and road-map for creating a superior consumer experience; one that focuses on the needs of people, not the medical-industrial complex. Based on his experience as a physician and healthcare leader, Zeev Neuwirth combines lessons from marketing and business with proven ways to innovate. Anyone dissatisfied with the current state of healthcare will enjoy the book, and that's most of us!*

Robert Pearl MD

former CEO of The Permanente Medical Group & former president of The Mid-Atlantic Permanente Medical Group

author of *Mistreated: Why We Think We're Getting Good Healthcare and Why We're Usually Wrong*

If you're trying to win in a "status quo" healthcare game, this is a must read. Zeev will convince you it's time to change course. The current system isn't just inefficient and expensive, it's inhumane. As leaders in healthcare, we owe something more to all Americans. If you're already trying to break the status quo, Zeev provides a step-by-step guide and invaluable real-world examples from which to learn and be inspired.

Chris Chen MD

CEO, ChenMed

REFRAMING HEALTHCARE

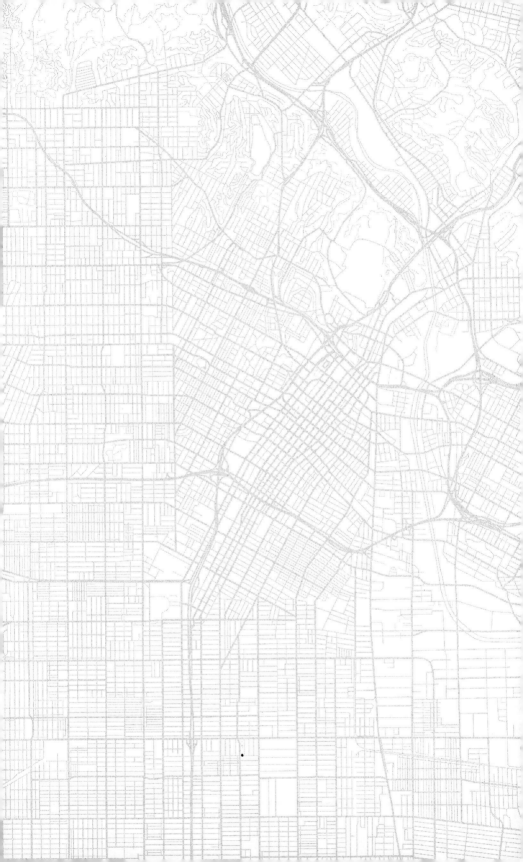

REFRAMING HEALTHCARE

A ROADMAP FOR
CREATING DISRUPTIVE CHANGE

ZEEV E. NEUWIRTH, MD

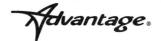

Copyright © 2019 by Zeev E. Neuwirth.

All rights reserved. No part of this book may be used or reproduced in any manner whatsoever without prior written consent of the author, except as provided by the United States of America copyright law.

Published by Advantage, Charleston, South Carolina.
Member of Advantage Media Group.

ADVANTAGE is a registered trademark, and the Advantage colophon is a trademark of Advantage Media Group, Inc.

Printed in the United States of America.

10 9 8 7 6 5 4 3 2 1

ISBN: 978-1-59932-898-0
LCCN: 2019934917

Book design by Megan Elger.

This publication is designed to provide accurate and authoritative information in regard to the subject matter covered. It is sold with the understanding that the publisher is not engaged in rendering legal, accounting, or other professional services. If legal advice or other expert assistance is required, the services of a competent professional person should be sought.

Advantage Media Group is proud to be a part of the Tree Neutral® program. Tree Neutral offsets the number of trees consumed in the production and printing of this book by taking proactive steps such as planting trees in direct proportion to the number of trees used to print books. To learn more about Tree Neutral, please visit **www.treeneutral.com**.

Advantage Media Group is a publisher of business, self-improvement, and professional development books and online learning. We help entrepreneurs, business leaders, and professionals share their Stories, Passion, and Knowledge to help others Learn & Grow. Do you have a manuscript or book idea that you would like us to consider for publishing? Please visit **advantagefamily.com** or call **1.866.775.1696**.

This book is dedicated to my mother—Ruth Chaimovitz Neuwirth.

Thank you for teaching me to think for myself, to speak up for what I believe in, and to listen to others with an open heart and mind.

I owe so much of this book to you.

TABLE OF CONTENTS

INTRODUCTION xiii

THE PROBLEM

CHAPTER 1 1
"Houston, We Have a Problem"

THE SOLUTION

CHAPTER 2 21
The Reframe Roadmap

CHAPTER 3 45
The Marketing Mindset

REBRANDING

CHAPTER 4 79
Rebranding

CHAPTER 5 97
Rebranding Primary Care

REDESIGNING

CHAPTER 6 121
Redesigning

CHAPTER 7 137
Principles of Redesign

REORGANIZING

CHAPTER 8 159
Reorganizing

CHAPTER 9 179
The Disruptive Potential of Reorganizing

NEW REFRAMES

CHAPTER 10 197
Game-Changing Trends

CHAPTER 11 221
The "Social Determinants of Health" Reframe

EPILOGUE 243
A Call to Action

ACKNOWLEDGMENTS 251

REFERENCES 261

ADDITIONAL RESOURCES 277

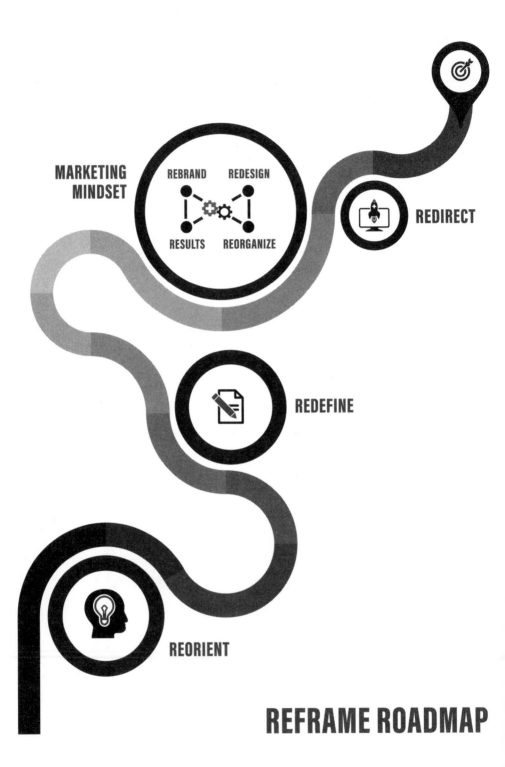

MARKETING
MINDSET

REBRAND   REDESIGN

RESULTS   REORGANIZE

REDIRECT

REDEFINE

REORIENT

REFRAME ROADMAP

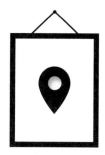

INTRODUCTION

ALL OF US deserve access to affordable, high quality, customer-oriented healthcare. Yet, despite all the world-class expertise, technology, cutting edge research, well-intentioned efforts, and profound resources within our healthcare system, we continue to experience healthcare outcomes that fall far short of what we would like to believe. Healthcare outcomes in the US are, at best, mediocre compared to other developed nations in the world. But, we have the ability—right now—to unleash the tremendous value that's currently locked up in our healthcare system, and to deliver the type of healthcare we all expect and deserve.

IT'S TIME to do something different—very different. One of the biggest limitations to date has been our own constrained thinking. We must change not just *what* we think and do, but *how* we think and do. And we must follow through. We must take these new ideas and transpose them into desirable, feasible, and sustainable endeavors and then actually implement them.

THIS BOOK offers a step-by-step guide on how we can do things very differently in order to enact the much-needed changes to healthcare. We can make healthcare easier, more affordable, more effective, safer, and more respectful of its consumers. The *Reframe Roadmap* that I share in this book has been distilled from nearly three decades of hands-on experience as well as hundreds of hours of interviews with cutting edge healthcare leaders and entrepreneurs. It's also supported by the past dozen years I've spent working as a physician executive and innovator, to redesign and reorganize healthcare delivery.

This book is a guide for leaders. It's written for those individuals who have the influence, capabilities, and authority to positively impact healthcare in a profound way. It's directed at leaders who don't just want to play the game, but to those who want to change the game; leaders who aren't seeking incremental improvements, but instead, transformative ones. It's written for boards and senior leadership teams who want to position their organizations and their communities to be part of creating a better healthcare.

These leaders belong to three main categories: (1) *leaders of organizations that are current stakeholders* in healthcare such as hospital systems, provider groups, healthcare insurance companies, employers, pharmaceutical and device manufacturers, as well as federal and state-level health service agencies; (2) *leaders of organizations that are new entrants* to the field of healthcare, including retailers, online retailers, and digital-tech, analytics, and telecom corporations that are rapidly becoming significant players in the $3.5 trillion US healthcare industry—as well as the thousands of smaller start-up entrepreneurs—and (3) *leaders of consultancies, vendor organizations, patient activist coalitions, medical associations, and professional societies.*

This book will inform these leaders about: 1) why numerous attempts to transform healthcare have failed over the past few decades; 2) the underlying forces driving the trends and changes in healthcare; and 3) the steps we need to take in order to assure that we transform the current approach into one that is consumer-centric, community-oriented, value-laden, and sustainable for our children and grandchildren.

Although this book is targeted at leaders, it's also written for any individual who has ever been frustrated, frightened, angered, or harmed by the healthcare system and who simply wants to understand it better.

Why I Wrote This Book

I once heard a comment by Reid Hoffman, the founder of LinkedIn. He used the term "frustrated awe." This phrase really captures my sense of American healthcare. I've always been in awe of healthcare, and I've always been deeply frustrated with it. I'm passionate about the state of US Healthcare for both personal and professional reasons. I have spent three decades in the healthcare system doing my best to deliver and support others in delivering the best medical care. The primary focus and thrust of my entire career has been to transform healthcare. This began with my career as a physician and medical educator, carried through in my work as a physician manager, and then as a process improvement innovator and quality officer. This remained my focus during the years I spent as an executive responsible for thousands of providers and it continues to describe my present role in helping manage the care of large populations of patients.

Throughout this journey, I have been:

- *Appalled and angered by the way that patients and their families are treated within the system.* Too often have I observed the lack of respect and dignity accorded to patients—the absence of empathy and understanding. In our healthcare system, patients have endured a lack of basic customer service and of transparency for too long. They've been exposed to suboptimal quality and uncoordinated care—care driven by volume over value, profit over purpose, and mechanics over meaning.

- *Shocked and disturbed by the way the system makes it difficult for dedicated professionals and staff to do the right thing on behalf of their patients.* I've always been in awe of the bright, passionate, hard-working, mission-driven professionals who take on the weighty responsibility of providing medical care daily; and who continue to sacrifice much for that privilege of providing care, even after years of being beaten down by the system.

- *Frustrated and frightened by the experience of being a patient, and even more so, of being a parent, spouse, or other close family member of a patient.* The current system is not built around its customers; it's built around itself and its own needs.

- *Encouraged and inspired by the extraordinary life-enhancing and life-saving work that I am privileged to witness, hear, or read about each day in the system.* I am in awe of the expertise, patience, and kindness of healthcare professionals and staff. Every day they demonstrate the nobility, meaningfulness, and importance of this endeavor.

- *Excited by and enthusiastic about what healthcare can become.* This includes the potential for people to be healthy in ways that go far beyond what we do today. There's a quote by noted author William Gibson: "The future is already here, it's just not very evenly distributed." I have always sought real-life, sustainable examples of what healthcare can become; rather than rely on optimism, idealism, or theory. I fully realize that we can treat patients and their families better; support our providers and staff better; collaborate and innovate better; and incorporate science, technology, and empathy so much better. What's required is *courageous leadership and a roadmap*. Over the past thirty years, I've learned that I'm not wired to settle for proximal change. I am wired to assist and support others in creating remarkably better experiences and outcomes.

I wrote this book because of, and for, the tens of thousands of patients and families I've treated or witnessed being treated, and the thousands of providers and administrators I've worked with all along the way. I wrote this book because of the good, the bad, and the ugly that I've both participated in and observed. I know that I could have done much better and that there were moments where I lost my conviction and hope; moments of fatigue and frustration; moments where I fell far short of my professional aspiration, goals, and credo; and moments where ego and self-interest got the better of me.

I wrote this book because I needed to. I needed to share what I've been experiencing and studying; because I see us continuing to do the same things over and over again while expecting different results. I needed to, because I believe we can unlock the profound potential that is currently bound within the constraints of our thinking and the current context. I needed to, because I can now see how reframing healthcare can make things so much better for providers, and more importantly, for healthcare consumers and their families. I needed to, because the approach I've distilled deserves to be placed in much more capable hands than mine. It needs to be placed in the hands of super-conscious and super-competent leadership in organizations across the country and across the world—the policy leaders, business leaders, operational leaders, finance leaders, medical leaders, and technology leaders who are and will be creating a new healthcare.

I wrote this book because I didn't want to look back ten or twenty years from now and wish I had shared this roadmap with others. I believe that the broad deployment and iteration of this reframe approach can alleviate tremendous suffering in the years to come, and I would not forgive myself if I hadn't at least attempted to share it widely.

There is one other critically important reason why I wrote this book. What I have finally realized, after decades of speaking up within organizations, is that there is precious little space, time, and attention within healthcare organizations—or even within medical societies or conferences—to create and sustain a meaningful dialogue focused on the topic of "creating a new healthcare system." Within healthcare, we are not collectively building in the time and are not providing the appropriate attention to this critically important issue of "reframing" healthcare delivery, despite the generally accepted understanding that this is what we must do. The vast majority of people within healthcare—providers, staff, managers, and even executives—do not feel heard, on this account. I can't begin to tell you how many times I've heard even senior leaders describe that they're not able to voice their true beliefs or work to direct healthcare delivery in the ways they believe it should head.

So I wrote this book, launched my podcast, and have been facilitating board level retreats, in large part to create the space and time for a different dialogue—a dialogue in which people can give voice to their true beliefs about healthcare delivery. A dialogue in which people can focus their primary attention, and intention, on the right things to do for their patients, their customers, and their communities—a dialogue in which people can reconnect with their purpose and their passion for serving humanity. This is not an idealistic quest. It's a very concrete and real dilemma for those of us who bear the tremendous responsibility to steward healthcare delivery.

As I discuss in the epilogue of this book, this is not a criticism of healthcare organizations or of the healthcare system. It's an observation. Sadly, I believe it's ubiquitous and I suspect that it's true in other industries as well. Again, please understand that this is not a criticism of our organizations or their leadership. I understand, firsthand, the daily pressures and responsibilities that sit on the shoulders of leaders as well as providers and staff in healthcare organizations. The daily work is all-consuming. It seems almost impossible to lift one's head up and have this different, forward-facing dialogue. That's why I wrote this book. That's why I host a podcast with successful leaders and entrepreneurs who are courageously building a new healthcare. And that's why I'm speaking with senior leadership teams and boards across the country—to create the space and time for this sort of dialogue, and to give the necessary attention to reframing healthcare.

Ultimately, I wrote this book, and am engaged in these other efforts, in order to humanize healthcare—humanize it for those who serve within the system and especially for those who are served by the system.

Why I Wrote This Book *Now*

There is a catalytic event that played a role in my actually sitting down to write this book. Four years ago, I—along with my brother, two sisters, and father—lost my mother. Ruth was in her early seventies and died in a hospital after a long, painful post-operative course, following a completely elective surgery for her arthritic hip. My mother was one of the hundreds of thousands of people who die avoidable, preventable deaths each year in the US healthcare system. She died from a bacterial infection in her bowels, *Clostridium dificile*, and the subsequent septic shock that ensued. The tragedy is that this infection could have been prevented by her providers and staff simply washing their hands in between caring for patients as well as avoiding the prescribing of unnecessary antibiotics. Now, I've been a health-care process improvement and quality improvement professional for many years, and I understand that it's the system, not the individuals, that are the root cause of most problems. But the truth is that there were many other preventable mishaps along the way that contributed to my mother dying, instead of leaving the hospital with a new hip.

My mother's death was not, however, *the* reason I wrote this book; perhaps it was one of the final straws. For the past few years, I have increasingly wondered: How many *hundreds of thousands of people* have to die unnecessary deaths in this country before we decide to act differently? How many *tens of millions of people* in this country have to go without adequate healthcare? How many *hundreds of millions* of people in this country have to be frustrated and harmed by a system that does not optimally support and promote their health?

My career has been focused on quality, safety, process improve-ment, care redesign, and patient-centered care. I have been formulat-ing this "reframe" approach for over a decade. In the aftermath of my mother's death, I decided that I would do what she had encouraged me to do—to speak up and share my perspective, my take on what we should do and how we should do it.

So, within a year after Ruth's passing, I began speaking at sympo-siums and conferences about this idea of *reframing healthcare*. People hearing me speak asked for something in writing to take back to their colleagues. So, I began the intensive research for what was initially an article, but which quickly turned into a book project. The additional research and interviews I conducted led me to launch a podcast to share the various ways in which both successful entrepreneurs and legacy leaders were rebranding, redesigning, and reorganizing healthcare. The inspiring, heroic journeys that I've posted on the podcast over the past couple of years as well as the encouraging feedback from listeners and the audiences that I've spoken with in person have all further fueled the production of this book. I wrote this book because I had to. I wrote it *now*, because I could not stand by any longer without taking the action that I believe is necessary to make things different and better.

How This Book is Organized

The book starts with an articulation of the problem facing the entire system of healthcare in the United States so that we have a shared, baseline understanding of why reframing healthcare is so critically important. In the second section, I introduce the concept of *Reframing Healthcare* by explaining what it means to reframe and why reframing is the most all-encompassing and essential transformative process that must be accomplished in healthcare delivery today. There are three main steps to the **Reframe Roadmap**: *Reorienting* our thinking; *Redefining* the problem given that new orientation; and *Redirecting* our strategies, tactics, and resources. In the second section, I also introduce one of the most fundamental parts of the Reframe Roadmap—what I've labelled the "Marketing Mindset." The steps of the *Marketing Mindset* are: *Rebranding, Redesigning,* and *Reorganizing* for *Results*. The following three sections of the book are devoted to an introductory explanation and illustration of the steps of the *Marketing Mindset*. In the last section of the book, we'll explore a couple of game-changing trends in healthcare that occur within the context of the Marketing Mindset. And we'll conclude with what I consider to be another fundamental reframe of our time—a focus on the so-called, "*Social Determinants of Health*."

If you read or remember nothing else from this Introduction, please make it this one point: This book was not written simply to enhance understanding. It was written to catalyze action. It is a guide for leaders and leadership teams who are interested in and capable of taking immediate, game-changing action—not only to improve healthcare, but to transform it. It is a roadmap, a Reframe Roadmap, for creating positive, humanistic, and disruptive change.

One last comment before we begin this journey. If you are a provider, support staff, or an administrator at any level within healthcare—if you work in the healthcare system in any capacity—I want to express my deeply felt appreciation for what you do. This book is not intended as a critique. It's an empathetic and appreciative guide intended to support you in radically improving this most amazing service to humanity.

Respectfully,
Zeev E. Neuwirth, MD

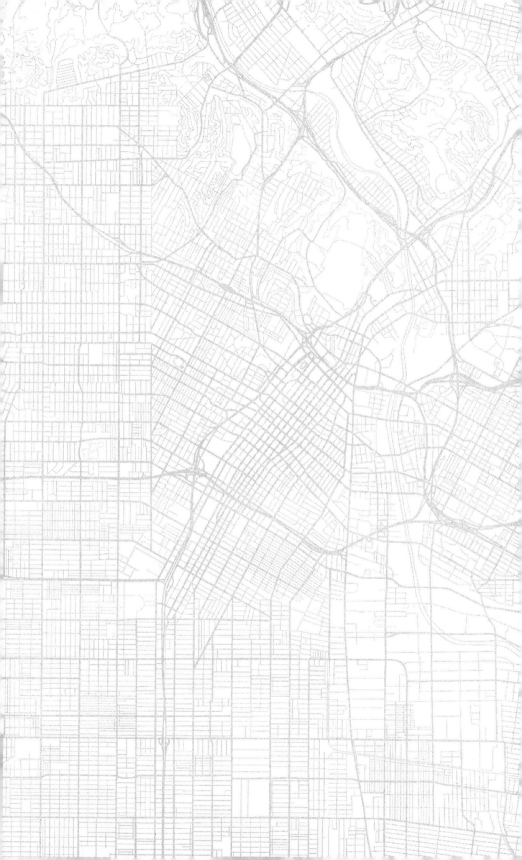

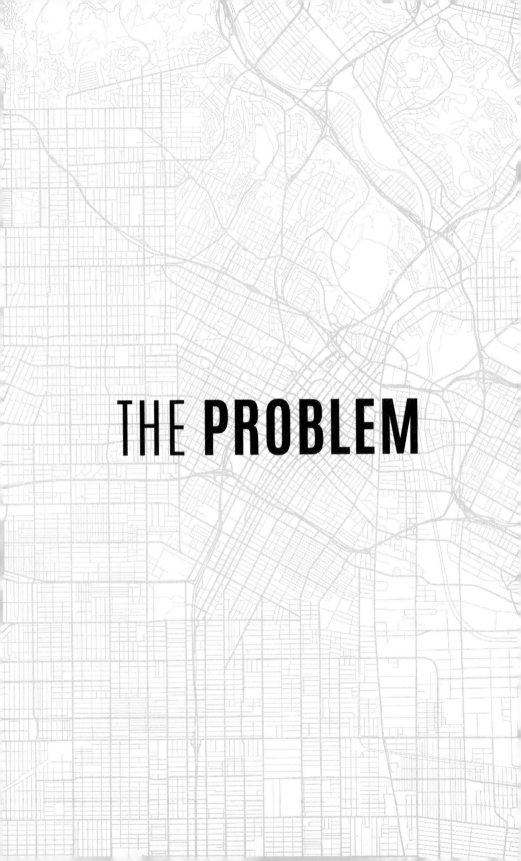

THE **PROBLEM**

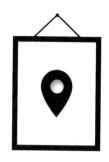

CHAPTER 1

"HOUSTON, WE HAVE A PROBLEM"

The vast majority of Americans believe that we have the best healthcare system in the world, and there isn't a shred of evidence that demonstrates that to be the case.

—Robert Pearl, MD (former CEO of the Permanente Medical Group & Mid-Atlantic Permanente Group of Kaiser Permanente)

Have you ever felt stuck repeating the same scenario over and over? After thirty years in healthcare, sitting in meeting after meeting, I have realized that the whole system of healthcare has been trapped in a "Groundhog Day" moment.

Those of you who recall the 1993 movie, *Groundhog Day*, with Bill Murray, will remember that he was stuck reliving the same day. He woke up every morning, hit that alarm clock, and was forced to repeat the same series of events, over and over and over again.

I have held many roles in the healthcare world, not only as a physician, but as a manager and executive. I've begun to have an increasing number of "Groundhog Day" moments over the past few years of my career. About three years prior to this writing, I was in a meeting with a number of other physicians and administrators. We were discussing how to improve access to medical care. It was a familiar conversation, and with good reason. Access to medical care is a big problem. How do we create greater access, so people can be seen by a healthcare professional in a timely and efficient fashion? There are not enough doctors and appointments; there are not enough hours in the day and not enough days in the year to meet the medical needs of most populations, particularly when it comes to primary care access. There is just not enough capacity to get patients into the office to see their doctors and get the medical-care services we all agree are necessary.

As I participated in that particular meeting three years ago, I noticed a growing unease welling up inside me—a mix of frustration and déjà vu. The feeling that I had done this all before was overwhelming. "Wait a minute," I thought to myself, trying to understand the intense emotionality of the moment. "Haven't I been in this meeting before?" Just like that, I flashed back to a meeting I'd been in five years prior—none of the same people, but the same white coats and suits sitting around the table discussing the same exact topic. What made it viscerally uncomfortable was that it was almost the exact same conversation. We were recirculating the same problems and eerily similar solutions that had been discussed and implemented years before. A moment later, I was flooded with memories of meetings spanning at least a decade and a half—all of them focused on the issues of access and productivity, quality and efficiency. It felt just like Bill Murray made it look like in *Groundhog Day*; waking up each morning only to find that you're repeating the same day and series of events over and over again. It was my first—but, unfortunately, not my last—frustrating recognition of the "Groundhog Day" moment in healthcare; a moment we have been caught up in for decades.

The visceral realization I experienced that day—and all the other days—was both personal and professional. It was a frustration on behalf of other people and on behalf of the system of healthcare that bore significant responsibility for those other people's lives. How could we be having these same conversations, over and over again, with so much at stake? My increased frustration came from sensing that time was running out; and from the fact that there were other meetings being had that were not "Groundhog Day" moments. There were other conversations out there in which healthcare was truly being advanced. I knew one thing for sure: I wanted to be part of that movement. I also wanted my incredibly well-intentioned and brilliant colleagues to be part of that movement. But mostly, the pit in my stomach—emerging from years of frustration combined with a renewed sense of urgency and possibility—was about *patients*. I wanted to change their experience with the healthcare system and, in doing so, radically improve their health outcomes.

Around the same time as my first recognition of the "Groundhog Day" phenomenon, I ran across a cartoon that struck me as a visual metaphor for the dilemma in healthcare. In the cartoon, there are two young fish swimming along. They are greeted by a much older fish swimming in the other direction. The older fish stops, smiles and says to the two young fishes, "Hey there, how's the water today?" He swims on his way, not waiting for their response. One of the young fishes turns to the other with a blank expression and a shrug, and asks, "What the heck is water?" In reading this cartoon, I immediately identified with the older fish and the two younger ones as well.

"What the heck is water?" For the two younger fishes, water is all they've ever known, so they take it for granted, not even noticing that it's a thing—that it even exists. In some ways, we're like the young fishes; so deeply mired in the present milieu of healthcare that we don't even recognize it as a fundamental construct or environment or ecology. "How's the water today?" isn't a meaningful question for us, because we continue to swim in the construct without realizing it as such. We are swimming, so to speak, in a system, but we don't recognize its qualities, let alone that it could be something other than what it is. Now, the visual metaphor breaks down a bit here, because the two fish in the cartoon have no need to change or remove themselves from their ecology. But, we do! Our water needs changing. The understanding we miss, in my estimation, is that we have to change the fundamental waters we're swimming in if we are going to get out of the dire situation we find ourselves in. It's not enough to swim faster or better or to build new channels in our current waters. We need to change the water in some very fundamental ways. In a very simple sense, the entirety of this book is aimed at helping us to do that—introducing a new approach (the Reframe Roadmap) and a new orientation (the Marketing Mindset); as well as the corresponding comprehensive set of steps that will allow us to perceive the water as such, and to change our healthcare environment—significantly improving its quality and sustainability for all of us fishes.

For years, we've pinned our hope for transforming healthcare on one silver bullet after another. But these bullets have all been stuck within a particular tradition of thinking about how healthcare works and should work. The

> *For years, we've pinned our hope for transforming healthcare on one silver bullet after another.*

bottom line is that all the creative strategies, the brilliant tactics, and the technologic wizardry we've attempted for decades has not gotten us out of this dire situation, because our thinking is mired in the confining context of a legacy framework. This is a huge dilemma involving costs, transparency, experience, safety, quality, outcomes, efficiency, accessibility, and equity of care. The problem is so multifold that it's difficult to keep it brief. We will not find a winning solution if we stick with the same way of thinking. What I propose in this book is that if we are going to transcend the pitfalls of the current system, we must reframe our approach entirely and comprehensively.

> *We will not find a winning solution if we stick with the same way of thinking.*

Steve Jobs said that in order to "do different" you have to "think different." His "think different" marketing campaign, and iconic Apple 1997 television ad, featured divergent thinkers and doers who changed the world around them—people like Mahatma Ghandi, Pablo Picasso, Muhammad Ali, and Martin Luther King Jr. Jobs's narrative began, "Here's to the crazy ones, the misfits, the rebels, the troublemakers, the round pegs in the square holes … the ones who see things differently…"

The purpose of this first chapter is to create a shared understanding of what I mean by a "dire dilemma" in healthcare. Its purpose is to lay out the current reality in healthcare and make a case for what we must leave behind and *why* we need to leave certain things behind in order to build a new and better healthcare. The vast majority of this book isn't about critiquing the problems. It's about how to generate solutions by seeing things differently and then acting differently.

That said, we have to start with where we are today, and we have to confront reality head on.

Quality, Safety, and Trust

We've come to expect that consumer products and services come with a basic assurance of quality and safety. As in other industries, quality, safety, and trust in healthcare are paramount. When you stepped into your car this morning, or onto a bus or train, did you pause to wonder if it was safe to do so? Or if the milk or cream you poured into your coffee this morning was contaminated? How about on your last flight—did you consider whether the pilots and staff were trained well enough to safely deliver you to your destination? The answer, in most cases, is no. We have the expectation of quality and safety, so we trust the products and services of these industries, almost as a given. But is that also the case when we engage with our healthcare system? Do you, or more to the point, *should you* trust the healthcare system to deliver high quality, safe service? Let's look at some statistics.

It's been estimated that there are somewhere between two hundred thousand to four hundred thousand avoidable deaths that occur each year in the US healthcare system.[1] Think about that: two hundred thousand to four hundred thousand avoidable, preventable deaths each year. Extrapolating from that number, each and every day in the United States of America, five hundred to one thousand people die, not directly from their illness or trauma, but from health-care—the very system that's supposed to heal them.[2]

Let me ask you this: if every single day, two or three jets mal-functioned due to some quality or safety issue, fell out of the sky, and killed everyone on board, what do you think the public reaction would be? How would the government react? Would you get on a jet anytime soon, or allow your family members to do so?

In healthcare, we still haven't accomplished what we set out to do starting in the late 1980s and 1990s, which was to solve the significant, and consequential quality and safety problems. We have improved, thanks to the tremendous effort of the quality and safety movement in healthcare; but even now, avoidable deaths make US healthcare—the delivery system *itself*—the third or fourth leading cause of death in this country.[3]

The World Health Organization and Commonwealth Fund data informs us that the US ranks on the lower end, in terms of quality and safety outcomes—typically last, compared to other developed nations.[4] These include both morbidity and mortality statistics.[5] That is mind boggling! We are the wealthiest nation in the world, with the best and brightest minds and some of the most stable infrastructure. It's not that we're not investing in healthcare, because we are. In fact, the amount we invest outweighs all other countries by a wide margin.[6] And it also isn't for lack of trying. It's not like we've been ignoring quality and safety within our hospitals, emergency rooms, operating suites, delivery rooms, and medical offices. Yet, despite all our well-intentioned efforts, we still rank last in overall healthcare outcomes, compared to other developed nations around the globe.

> *The US ranks on the lower end in terms of quality and safety outcomes.*

Let's take a closer look at just a few specifics.

Our rate, on average, of controlling high blood pressure—the primary cause of strokes and heart attacks—is only around 50 percent. When it comes to antibiotic usage in this country, only about half of the prescriptions for antibiotics have any evidence-based support for their efficacy. Even more disturbing: 50 percent of the approximately 270 million antibiotic prescriptions in 2017 were prescribed inappropriately.[7] We continue to see obesity rates rise; thirty percent of our population can now be labeled obese. Diabetes has become an epidemic over the last few decades, to the extent that now, approximately 10 percent of the US population has diabetes, and another 30 percent of the population can be labelled prediabetic.

We don't have to look very far to see the most obvious example of a healthcare-related, or more precisely, healthcare-induced epidemic: opioid usage! The Centers for Disease Control (CDC) released data showing that, in 2016, more than sixty-four thousand people died of drug overdoses in the United States. That surpasses the total number of Americans who were killed in the Vietnam War. It surpasses the number of people who died from AIDS at the height of that epidemic. And these overdose numbers are increasing. From 2015 to 2016, there was a 21 percent increase in the number of overdose deaths, the vast majority (75 percent) of which were opioid overdoses. While the use of illegal drugs, such as heroin, makes up a part of that number, the majority of it, according to the experts, is due to medication-driven opioids such as oxycodone and fentanyl. In fact, whereas heroin-related deaths increased by 17 percent between 2015 and 2016, fentanyl-related deaths increased by 103 percent that same year. In other words, the bigger problem is inappropriately prescribed opioids, not street opioids.

Much has been written and more is being uncovered about the unethical politics and business dealings within our healthcare system that drove this epidemic. Much of it was unintended, at least on the provider side. I remember, as a practicing physician in the 1990s and early 2000s, that major pharmaceutical campaigns in healthcare centered around identifying pain, measuring pain, and treating pain with opioids like oxycodone. I remember the development of pain schedules and protocols. It was all in service of patient care, or so we believed.

We're now realizing that this epidemic is not going to end any time soon. It's going to go on for quite some time, because we've essentially caused generations of Americans to be plagued by addiction. One last stat on this account: although the US population makes up less than 5 percent of the world's population, we consume over 80 percent of the pain medications! Our American healthcare system has generated an epidemic of yet untold magnitude and misery.[8]

Feeling uncomfortable yet?

Cost

When it comes to healthcare, the US spends more than any other developed country—somewhere around $10,000 per year, per person. Given that cost, it should come as no surprise that almost 30 percent of Americans report having problems paying their medical bills; and of that 30 percent, over 70 percent have to cut back spending on food, clothing, or basic household items in order to pay for healthcare.[9]

Medical costs and health-insurance payments have been the leading cause of wage stagnation in our country. Even though wages are increasing, the hidden truth is that healthcare-benefit costs are increasing faster, so individuals and families are actually bringing home

Over 50 percent of the American public say they're worried that they won't be able to afford healthcare in the future.

less than they were before. Over 50 percent of the American public say they're worried that they won't be able to afford healthcare in the future. And they *should* be worried. We know that healthcare has been and continues to be a leading cause of individual and family bankruptcy. Even more disturbing, over 70 percent of people who file bankruptcy due to healthcare costs *have health insurance.*

Let's be clear: this isn't a problem of the uninsured or even the very poor in our country. This is a problem facing middle- and upper-class Americans as well. An October 2018 study by the Commonwealth Fund showed that for people with insurance who have had a serious medical condition or a course of hospital care, over one-third used up all or almost all of their savings; nearly a third were contacted by a collection agency; 21 percent were unable to pay for basic necessities like food or heat as a result of their medical expenses; 13 percent had to borrow money, get a loan, or put a second mortgage on their homes; and 4 percent had to declare personal or family bankruptcy.[10] Can you imagine that? One out of every twenty-five families who experience a serious medical condition have to declare bankruptcy as a result of the medical expense, and that's for *families who have health insurance!* For those without insurance, the situation is even more dire; nearly 60 percent use up all their savings and are contacted by a collection agency; and 50 percent are unable to pay for basic necessities like food, housing, or heat.[11]

The inexcusable and reprehensible burden of healthcare costs doesn't end with individuals and their families. Municipalities, towns, counties, and states also struggle to pay for healthcare. Just like households, they're diverting expenditures for other things, whether it be police, fire safety, roads and bridges, sewage, and— most importantly—education. In March 2018, the current senior administrator for the Centers for Medicare & Medicaid, Dr. Seema

Verma, articulated the situation accurately, "The system we have is unsustainable, and it cannot continue … because this increase in spending will continue to crowd out funding for other priorities, such as roads and schools, as well as national defense."[12]

Healthcare is also a major line-item concern for corporate America. Warren Buffet, one of the most successful and trusted financial investors and business minds of our time, summed it up by saying, "Healthcare is the hungry tapeworm of corporate America." Bill Gates, founder of Microsoft, and a software-industry icon, discussed the devastating dilemma that rising healthcare costs have placed on our society. In a 2011 Ted Talk, Gates described the terrible trade-off: either take care of the sick and elderly at the expense of the education of our children; or invest in the future of our children at the expense of providing medical care to the sick and elderly. Too many sectors of the US infrastructure are being shortchanged by the rising costs of healthcare—our future is being threatened by the rising costs of healthcare.

Far from slowing down, these costs are predicted to continue to rise for future generations—our children and our grandchildren. The World Health Organization issued a conservative estimate that millennials (those born between about 1978 and 1993) will spend somewhere between 50 and 70 percent of their lifetime earnings on healthcare costs. That's catastrophic. The staggering costs of healthcare are a national as well as global catastrophe.[13] According to the World Health Organization, overall global healthcare spending is expected to rise from about $8.4 trillion as of 2015 to $18.3 trillion in 2030. That's more than double in a fifteen-year period![14]

The undeniable point here is that the cost of healthcare is currently a crisis, and it's getting worse. Let's put aside, for a moment, the quality and safety issues we discussed earlier. If the cost issue isn't resolved, people won't even be able to *access* care, because it just won't be affordable. Experts have written about the potential for healthcare rationing in the future, but we don't have to look to the future. Healthcare rationing is already here. Significant racial and ethnic healthcare disparities exist, and they continue to get worse. We'll cover this later in the chapter on the social determinants of health.

We have a serious quality and safety problem in healthcare. We have an unsustainable and unjustifiable cost problem. And, the reality is that neither problem has been resolved or greatly improved by the changes and innovations we've introduced into healthcare in the past two or three decades.

Patient Satisfaction

For all the money we spend on healthcare (recall, on average, $10,000 per individual per year), it's astounding how little satisfaction we experience as consumers in the system. Customer satisfaction and loyalty within and across industries is measured by a standardized survey called the Net Promoter Score (NPS). It's a scale that goes from negative 100 to positive 100. Really strong brands, like Apple, typically score in the 70s or 80s, and industries with outstanding customer experience can even score in the 90s. So, how does healthcare do? As a sector, US healthcare generally scores in the teens or in the twenties on the NPS.

Public trust in the American healthcare system literally "crashed."

Another consumer score we can turn to for insight is called the Edelman Trust Barometer. It is a measure of comparative consumer experience—looking across industries and across countries. The

Barometer measures the "informed public's trust" for a given industry, in each country. In 2018, the Edelman Trust Barometer showed that public trust in the American healthcare system literally "crashed" twenty points from the year before—what they termed, "extreme trust loss." The only other country whose healthcare system saw a greater decline in public trust was Columbia. This US decline—a drop in the Edelman Trust Barometer score from 75 to 55—placed the US below the established "Trust" Zone. To provide some context, the US placed slightly better than Russia, which rated at 51, and Poland which was rated by its public at 48.[15]

The Gallup Poll has also been measuring public trust in "the medical system", with long-term results that parallel the Edelman Trust Barometer. According to the Gallup Poll, American public trust in the medical system has dropped from 74 percent in 1977 to 36 percent in 2018—an absolute decrease of 38 percent! Of the fifteen American institutions measured, no other has seen that large a drop. (The only other institution which has seen a similar decrease in trust is Congress.)[16] The 2018 Gallup Poll revealed that 80 percent of Americans were dissatisfied with the costs of healthcare, and nearly two-thirds rated healthcare as poor or fair. There was one aspect of healthcare with which Americans were more pleased: 55 percent rated quality positively.[17]

Another current barometer of the American public's dissatisfaction and concern with healthcare comes to us from election-polling sources. Pre-midterm election monitoring (June–August 2018) indicate that the #1 voter issue and concern on people's minds was healthcare. Healthcare costs, not surprisingly, topped these concerns.[18]

As someone who has worked for decades to enhance the patient experience, it is my estimation that the US healthcare system lags years, perhaps decades, behind other industries in terms of understanding and delivering a consumer-oriented experience. I've had this belief reinforced by consumer experts from the retail, dig-tech and entertainment industries. One example of this comes from Marcus Osborne, the VP of health transformation at Walmart, who shared his perspective in a recent interview: "We certainly respect consumers more than anybody in the healthcare industry does. Healthcare has to be about the consumer only. At the end of the day, physicians and hospitals exist to serve people." And the former chief of global consumer insight at Disney, Kevan Mabbutt, shared his perspective that: "consumerism is really very, very late to healthcare. I think healthcare has not been as competitive, by any stretch, in the U.S., as other industry sectors. And I think that's largely why it's been so un-consumer-centric and un-consumer-friendly."[19]

Paging "Dr. Burnt-Out"

Just as the experience of being a healthcare consumer within the current system is sorely lacking, it's no great shakes being a healthcare provider within the system either. The research informs us that, at the time of this writing, approximately half of the doctors in the US experience burn out, and the situation appears to be getting worse.

> *Approximately half of the doctors in the US experience burn out.*

The physicians, nurses, physician assistants, as well as other providers—who treat us every day in both low and high-risk situations—are the most critical creators of value in healthcare delivery. So, it's concerning, to say the least, that on average, *one out of every two* doctors is burnt out: demoralized, depersonalized, emotionally exhausted, or depressed.

The fact that such a significant percentage of providers score in the range of "burnt out" belies a much larger percentage, perhaps even the majority, who are disillusioned with the system and their profession.[20] What's terribly wrong with this picture is that these are individuals who are overwhelmingly mission-driven, dedicated, and resilient professionals—people who have committed their lives to be part of a challenging but meaningful profession—people who would love to love what they do and who want to sustain their dedication and service to others. But they face pressures and stress so great that they end up feeling demoralized and burnt out, or worse.

Approximately four hundred physicians commit suicide each year in the US, more than one per day, on average. The suicide rate among physicians is higher than for other professionals. For female physicians, it's particularly disturbing—about 250 percent higher than women in other professions.[21] From years of directly observing physicians behind closed exam room doors, I can unabashedly say that it's disturbing to watch burnt-out, stressed, and harried physicians trying to do the best they can under unacceptable and unsustainable circumstances. We've reduced healthcare to very pressured, transactional visits. Our fee-for-service, volume-driven payment and compensation models have reduced physicians and other providers to "visit vendors," particularly in primary care medicine. It's wrong, as much for practitioners as for the consumers of healthcare delivery.

One point I'd like to be clear about is that the people working in healthcare, including the administrators who are held accountable for the goals and metrics the system has imposed on them, are doing the best they can. These are superbly trained doctors, nurses, physician's assistants, techs, support staff, and administrators who bend over backwards daily to make the system work—and it clearly is back-breaking work. But, even so, that work is not translating into great customer experiences, optimal patient outcomes, or high-quality, cost-effective care.

Our Response, so Far, to the Problems in Healthcare

We've been attempting to solve these problems in healthcare for decades. We've thrown one solution after another at them, and each time, rather than helping solve problems, these "silver-bullet" solutions have made incremental improvements, if any; or have brought with them more challenges to be solved.

A few examples of incredibly well-intentioned attempted solutions have included years of organizational development work such as team building, leadership development, communication, and empathy skill building. Another set of examples includes the development of new tools and techniques, like those for measuring patient experiences, assessing quality care, or the transition to electronic health records. Please don't misunderstand me; I think it's a wonderful and critically important thing to measure quality and customer experience, and there is no question in my mind that the electronic health record (EHR) will prove to be a much more useful and reliable tool than hand-written notes stored on sheets of hard copy paper in office file cabinets. But right now, both the type and amount of data-retrieval, data-entry, and record-keeping associated with EHRs and quality metrics have greatly contributed to sub-optimizing care, to physician burn out, and to patient dissatisfaction. The current state of electronic medical records has, to some extent, devolved into a "check-the-box" mentality and a "garbage-in/garbage-out" situation.

Barbara McAneny, MD, (at the time of this writing, the president-elect of the American Medical Association), has commented that in no other profession is the most highly skilled and highly paid personnel forced to do what amounts to entry-level data work and filling out of forms.[22] Alex Azar, the current secretary for Health & Human Services commented on the present situation in a 2018 speech, "It's the patients who suffer when a provider spends more time reporting quality measures than delivering care."[23] Even Dr. Don Berwick, one of the most brilliant and impactful leaders of the healthcare quality and safety movement over the past four decades, comments on the unintended outcomes of mis-applying quality metrics, "…we're dealing with an insane amount of metrics that hospitals or clinicians deal with, and it impedes work. It doesn't help work… let's put measurement on a diet and use it for the purposes of learning and improvement, not as a tool in combat."[24]

Another category of attempts to solve our healthcare dilemma over the past two or three decades has been the process-improvement movement—TQM (Total Quality Measurement), Six Sigma, the "Lean" Toyota Production System, PDSA cycles, and so forth. While these approaches play a critically important role in obtaining and maintaining reliability, the belief that they would transform healthcare, or any other industry for that matter, has largely been abandoned. More recently, we've turned to the magic of virtual telehealth and digital technologies, chatbots, voice recognition, data clouds, pools and lakes, predictive analytics, machine learning, artificial intelligence, and ledger-based block chain algorithms. We're still relatively early-on in these latest trends, but decades

If we're looking for a technologic magic bullet to transform healthcare, we're most likely misguided in our thinking.

of experience and the wisdom of cutting-edge experts and entrepreneurs informs us that if we're looking for a technologic magic bullet to transform healthcare, we're most likely misguided in our thinking.

Another major attempted solution set has been payment and reimbursement, which we'll touch upon in chapter 8. And while payment reformation—that is, the move to value-based payment—is an absolutely necessary component of any progressive solution moving forward in healthcare delivery, it is, in and of itself, insufficient in transcending the current quagmire we find ourselves in. Numerous countries around the globe have transitioned to a capitated payment model but continue to experience profound problems in sustaining their healthcare system. More to come on this topic in chapters 8 and 9 on reorganizing healthcare.

My point here is that our development and deployment of these solutions to date have not been adequate, and they've not achieved their potential for greatly improving healthcare. But, even more to the point: while these approaches, techniques, and tools have tremendous potential for improving healthcare, they are not the solution for transforming it. It is my firm belief that these are all necessary, but none are sufficient—not even collectively—as long as we remain within the same framework of thinking and doing. As one colleague said to me a number of years ago, "You can reengineer the horse and buggy all you like, but at the end of the day, you still have a horse and buggy." Remember the insights from the likes of Steve Jobs—you can't solve fundamental problems with the same thinking that caused it. In order to really solve (or perhaps dis-solve) the access, cost,

> *In order to really solve the seemingly unsolvable problems in healthcare, we have to think and do differently—very differently.*

quality, safety, equity, and numerous other seemingly unsolvable problems in healthcare, we have to *think and do* differently—*very* differently.

I recently heard a phrase which captures the situation pithily and provides a very concrete and compelling metaphor for why we need to reframe healthcare. It's somewhat similar to the fish cartoon message I referenced earlier. The phrase is, "you can't read the label of the jar you're in..." We need an effective, systematic, replicable, and sustainable approach to getting outside of the jar and reconstituting what's in it. And that's what the Reframe Roadmap is about.

Again, I hope I've made it clear that I would not recommend we discard or abandon any of the approaches, technologies, or solutions mentioned. I want to restate and emphasize that, in and of themselves, these are not transformative solutions. They're important and necessary, but not sufficient. They're not the resolutions to our biggest dilemmas—unless and until they become part of a bigger-picture shift in how we think about healthcare and health; unless and until they become part of a major healthcare reframe.

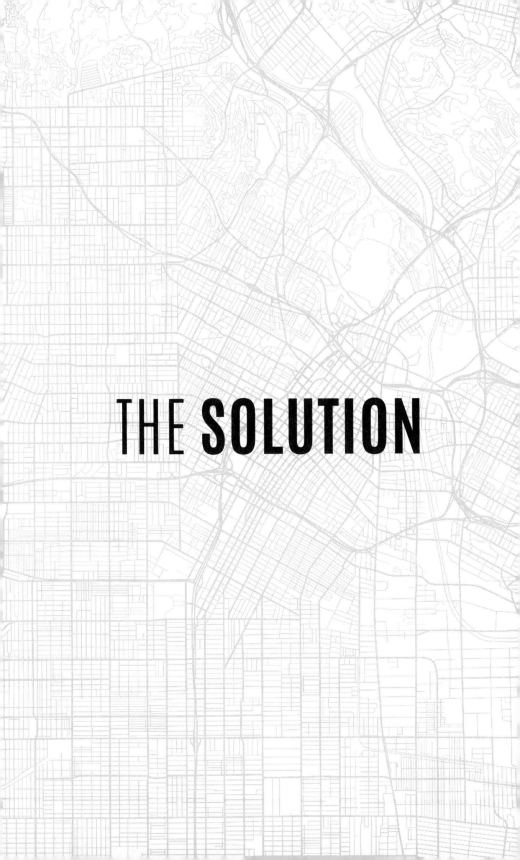

THE SOLUTION

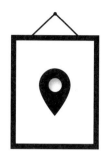

CHAPTER 2

THE REFRAME ROADMAP

(WE CAN'T JUST FIX HEALTHCARE)

When the business world encounters an intractable management problem, it's a sign that there isn't yet a satisfactory theory for what's causing the problem, and under what circumstances it can be overcome.

—Clayton Christensen, professor at Harvard Business School

As we've just discussed, the design of our healthcare system is not aligned to the needs of healthcare consumers nor to the needs of healthcare practitioners. Decades of attempts to fix the system haven't succeeded, and although each fix has been effective in some way, the system remains broken.

The design of our healthcare system is not aligned to the needs of healthcare consumers nor to the needs of healthcare providers.

Our situation in healthcare reminds me of another cartoon I recently came across, of the biblical Jews standing in the Sinai desert. In front of them is a map of the desert posted on a banner. It's a large "you are here" type of map, the kind of map you might see in an amusement park or in a retail shopping mall. On the map is a squiggly line that goes around and around, leading nowhere. The only landmark besides "you are here" is "Egypt," the place they came from. It's clear that they know where they've been, but they don't know where they're going or how to get there.

This cartoon resonates deeply with my sense of the current situation in healthcare. We have been wandering around, lost in the "healthcare dilemma" desert for decades. The biblical Jews were forced to wander for forty years. But, have you ever wondered why it was forty years? The Sinai desert doesn't take anywhere close to forty years to cross, even by foot. To provide some context: the distance between Cairo and Jerusalem, which extends beyond the dimensions of the Sinai desert, is only about 265 miles, as the crow flies. There are numerous explanations for why the journey required this length of time. One explanation I've heard is that the biblical Jews needed time to rid themselves of their previous way of thinking, to develop and adopt a new mindset in order to cross into the promised land and create a new society and culture. They needed to (in my verbiage) *reframe* their perspective. If one looks at archetypal journey stories from other religions and cultures, such as the classic Greek and Roman mythologies, a similar theme emerges. In order to transform, there has to be a fundamental shift in perception. Joseph Campbell, the renowned scholar, taught us that, in order to be completed, the hero's journey—be it an individual or an entire people—requires a transformation in how we perceive ourselves and the world around us. Along similar lines, the understanding I've come to, through years of participation and studied observation, is that a fundamental require-ment for us to move into a new era—a transformed healthcare era—is a reframed set of perspectives. I believe that we have the opportu-nity and the ability to end our wandering, and that a comprehensive reframe would offer us a map out of the "healthcare dilemma" desert. Conversely, if we don't reframe our perspectives, we could continue to experience "Groundhog Day" moments three, five, ten, perhaps even twenty years from now. We must not only be aware of the waters we're swimming in; we must find a fundamentally different way of perceiving, thinking, and acting. The Reframe Roadmap and Marketing Mindset that I will introduce you to in this book are more than problem-solving tools or process-optimizing techniques. These are guides for transforming how we view our situation—guides that enable us to solve and/or dis-solve the multiple problems we've been grappling with for decades. As I've learned along the way, you can't reengineer yourself out of a fundamentally flawed design. Allow me to share a bit more on this account.

In 1997, Michael Hammer and James Champy co-authored a book entitled *Reengineering the Corporation: A Manifesto for Business Revolution*. To give you a sense of the importance of this work in business management, Mr. Hammer was recognized by *Business Week* as one of the top four management gurus of the time. He was a leader in the major business movement of that era—what one might call the "era of reengineering." I was, in full disclosure, caught up in that era as much as anyone else. In fact, I initiated and led a multi-year reengineering campaign from 2005 to 2009 (using the "Lean" Toyota Production System) in the provider group where I served at the time, Harvard Vanguard Medical Associates. I also initiated another multi-year Lean initiative at Carolinas Healthcare System (now known as Atrium Health), in 2012. As I alluded to in chapter 1, I had thrown myself into this solution set with the hope that it could be the catalyst to dig us out of the dilemmas we faced in healthcare delivery. At least, that was the promise, and there was good reason to believe it. But sometime during the fourth year of our deploying the reengineering approach across the expanse of Harvard Vanguard Medical Associates, I began to suspect that while Lean and Six Sigma were powerful techniques for process improvement and optimization, they were not a tool kit for innovation or transformational change.

Interestingly enough, at about the same time that I was coming to this understanding, a series of articles were being published in the business-management literature, in journals such as the *Harvard Business Review*, which substantiated my experience with reengineering. These publications and studies, which continue to be published up until the time of this writing, revealed quantified evidence that reengineering was not delivering on its expected return on investment. The reengineering approach had been adopted in the US in the 1980s and 1990s across a wide swath of industries including automobile manufacturers, telecommunications, consumer electronics, pharmaceuticals, banking, and the airline industry. A significant percentage of Fortune 500 and Fortune 100 Companies—well-known brands such as Motorola, GE, 3M, Dupont, Honda, Toyota, Bank of America, British Airlines, Honeywell, and Johnson & Johnson— had rigorously resourced and deployed Six Sigma, the Lean Toyota Production System, or some combination as a bedrock of their management approach. After a decade or so, however, these companies and their respective industries were not realizing the financial gains they had anticipated, and some were falling behind in being innovative leaders within their sector. To be fair, reengineering has resulted in benefits for some organizations. But I think it's safe to say that the major industries, including healthcare, have come to realize the limitations as well as the unintended consequences of reengineering.

While the reengineering tool kit will likely continue to be a necessary component for efficiency, continuous improvement, and reliability, I've come to realize that we must move into a new era—an era of reframing. If the providers and distributors of healthcare and of health-inducing products and services are going to meaningfully advance and elevate the health outcomes for individuals, families, communities, corporations, and this country, we're going to have to do much more than simply continue to reengineer and/or enhance our technologies. We're going to have to fundamentally change (some would even suggest abandon) the overall approach to healthcare as it's currently constructed. However you'd like to conceptualize or describe the transformation in healthcare, we're going to, as other industries have done, shift from an era of reengineering to an era of reframing.

> *We're going to, as other industries have done, shift from an era of reengineering to an era of reframing.*

What is a "Reframe?"

Let's look at what it means to reframe, and why we need a reframe to transcend the current dilemmas in which healthcare is trapped.

The first thing to understand about my approach to reframing is that it's not about hypothesizing or predicting some future potential or the next megatrend. It's not at all about what might happen. Instead, it's about discerning what has already occurred, what is happening now, and what is clearly emerging as an essential, underlying foundational pattern of reformation. At its core, it's a changed way of perceiving problems and goals as well as acting on that perception. It's an approach that requires us to understand our situation from a different perspective in order to shake ourselves free from being stuck. The best explanation of reframing that I've encountered comes from Peter Drucker, who reoriented our understanding of modern management and set the conceptual foundation for how most of us currently work in corporations. Many consider him to be the "founder" of modern management. He created concepts like the "knowledge worker," "management to goals," "outsourcing," "decentralization," and other constructs that we now take for granted. Drucker spoke of theory as coming from the reality of our practices:

> Intellectuals and scholars tend to believe that ideas come first, which then lead to new political, social, economic, and psychological realities. This does happen, but it is the exception. As a rule, theory does not precede practice. Its role is to structure and codify already proven practice. Its role is to convert the isolated and "atypical" from exception to "rule" and "system," and therefore into something that can be learned and taught and, above all, into something that can be generally applied. [25]

In a similar way to how Drucker's approach to theory transformed management, I believe that reframing can transform healthcare. In keeping with Drucker's approach, I didn't create the idea of a healthcare reframe. Instead, I observed it, distilled it, and tested it against dozens of examples. This notion of reframing is something that I've observed already in action, in healthcare as well as in other industries, and even in facets of people's lives, both professional and personal.

Life-Altering Reframes

Drucker was famous for bringing into his management theory concepts from history, sociology, psychology, philosophy, popular culture, and religion. Similar to Drucker, I've taken an interdisciplinary approach to my explanation of reframing. So, as we begin to think about the healthcare reframe, I want to share with you the story of a man who serves as a remarkable example of the nature and power of the reframe: Robert Lang. Lang was an engineer and physicist specializing in laser optics.[26] He earned his PhD at Cal Tech with a doctoral dissertation titled, *Semiconductor Lasers: New Geometries and Spectral Properties.* Lang's brilliant career included working in NASA's jet-propulsion lab, generating dozens of publications and patents, and serving as the editor in chief of the IEEE *Journal of Quantum Electronics.*

Lang's resume might lead you to believe that his professional accomplishments would remain within the realm of aeronautical physics and engineering. However, at the age of forty, Lang left a very successful and promising career to pursue his lifetime passion for origami. Yes, you read it right—origami, the Japanese art of folding a single piece of paper to create new forms. Origami is a tradition that is centuries old and is now practiced worldwide. Lang had been working on origami since he was a child, in part because he was bored in school, and this gave him a creative outlet.

As an adult, Lang started to create computer algorithms that would solve these complex folding problems, and he used laser technology to crease the paper. He would spend up to months developing these mathematical algorithms and then hours folding his projects. As you might imagine, this was a radical transformation, not just an incremental improvement in existing origami practices. Prior to

Lang, the best origami experts in the world could fold a piece of paper somewhere around thirty times. With the aid of his algorithms and computer programs, Lang was able to fold a single, uncut piece of paper up to one hundred times. This allowed him to create shapes that were so creative and sophisticated that they were essentially origami *sculptures.*[27]

How can a research physicist completely switch gears and go from working in jet propulsion and semiconductors to folding paper? I think this story directly illustrates the idea of the reframe. Lang took his background in physics, computer science, mathematics and engineering, and essentially reframed the approach to origami; not only mastering but entirely reshaping a discipline that had been around for centuries. He looked at this creative paper folding much differently than it had been looked at for hundreds of years.

What is so important about what Lang did and what are the take-away lessons here? He *reoriented* the story, which was no longer about folding pieces of paper with hands, eyes, and the power of an individual's mind. He shifted origami into a matter of applied mathematics and physics. He *redefined* the challenge. Folding problems became math problems, algorithmic problems, and pro-gramming problems. Then he *redirected* concrete strategies, tactics, and resources toward that end. As far as I know, no other origami expert in the world was doing what he was doing. Lang wasn't just improving upon an existing pattern or approach. He was creating a brand-new framework.

Robert Lang is exceptional not just in his transformation of origami, but because he is one of a very few people who has reframed multiple fields. On the basis of his work in origami, his space-industry colleagues approached him. They had a challenge with their immense telescopes and solar panels, some of them the size of a football field, that they deployed in space to collect images or solar energy. This large equipment had to be fitted with incredible precision and efficiency into small payloads in order to be propelled into outer space. Lang helped his colleagues *reframe* their challenge as a *folding* problem, so they could engineer the panels and telescopes to fold into the payload and then, once in space, unfold, unharmed, to collect energy and images.

This double reframe, in itself, was remarkable, but Lang's story doesn't stop there. He applied the folding reframe not only to the space industry, but also to the healthcare industry. There are plenty of folding problems in medicine. Intravascular stents, for example, used in cardiology and vascular surgery, are placed in arteries through thin hollow wires. When deployed, they hold open arteries that were clogged. In order to be inserted, they have to be folded into a very small package, and in order to work, they need to be able to be opened in arteries, or in the heart. Lang reframed a medical-device challenge by assisting the industry in how to fold stents and heart valves so they could be more effectively and safely released in patients.

All of these reframes in multiple industries came from one research scientist practicing origami. Lang's story vividly illustrates the sheer magnitude and power of what could be accomplished when a different perspective is brought to bear. Notice that Lang's reframes came from his everyday practice; practicing origami, physics, mathematics, and computer programming. Lang's reframes were about bringing together different traditions and perspectives. His training as a scientist enabled him to bring scientific tools to the practice of origami. His training in origami enabled him to bring both traditional and new paper-folding techniques to the space and healthcare industries.

The Necessity of a Roadmap

Without question, Lang has a brilliant mind, but I wouldn't want you to think that I'm recommending we wait around for the Langs of the world to reframe our problems in healthcare. What I've attempted to share in this book—stemming from years of speaking with and observing leaders, innovators, and entrepreneurs, and trying to understand how they see and solve problems—is a guideline. I've labelled it the Reframe Roadmap. It's a set of steps to support leaders and practitioners in *reorienting* and *redefining* their problems, in order to devise a *redirected* strategic course that allows for significant, positive systemic change.

For the few Langs of this world, a roadmap may not be required. But for most of us, a set of guidelines is required to assist us in reframing our situation or in helping others reframe the situation. There are numerous examples, largely from the military and from survival-psychology case studies demonstrating that when placed in harsh, high-stress, or disorienting situations, humans require a roadmap—a set of steps to assess and view the situation that allow them to take action so they can get out of those situations alive.

> A set of guidelines is required to assist us in reframing our situation.

John Leach is a psychologist who spent years researching people's decision-making in survival situations, such as being lost in the wilderness or experiencing a plane crash in remote regions. In studying what happens to people under these conditions, Leach has developed what he calls the "10-80-10 rule."[28] Ten percent of people in survival situations react hysterically; their behavior is so irrational that it is actually harmful to themselves and the others around them. These

10 percent are the ones who are most likely to perish, even in situations in which they objectively ought to survive. The vast majority, 80 percent of people, go into shock and sort of resign themselves to the situation. They are in a homeostatic mode. The remaining 10 percent of people react calmly and rationally and are most likely to survive and help others survive, even in surprisingly dire situations.

I suspect that some of you are nodding your heads thinking, "That's a great metaphor for what it feels like" to be working in healthcare or in other industries experiencing high-stress, disorienting situations; or even what it can sometimes feel like to be a patient. In the healthcare work environment, it does often feel like we're lost in the wilderness (recall the cartoon of the wandering biblical Jews)—just trying to survive in harsh, isolating, and stressful conditions; facing challenges that are constantly shifting. It can seem like we're always trying to understand the rules of the jungle and that there is no rescue or respite in sight, no guide to help us find a safe haven.

Recalling the statistics we cited in chapter 1, a significant percentage of providers and staff across the country are shell-shocked. Most people in healthcare who are at the front lines of care delivery can't even lift their heads up long enough to discover, let alone appreciate, a potential solution. According to Leach, 80 percent of individuals will react that way—not moving forward or looking for a way out, or for a way to improve the situation. Healthcare managers end up focusing a lot of effort on the extreme 10 percent who respond with behaviors that are downright caustic and harmful, those naysayers who won't quit or leave and who poison the morale for everyone. As Leach points out, this, too, is a natural phenomenon in survival-mode group psychology.

All told, according to Leach, 90 percent of people in survival situations will either do nothing or make the situation worse. The military has observed and understood the devastating consequences of this phenomenon. As a result, military leaders, for decades, have been purposefully developing and deploying survival guidelines—step-by-step approaches, and now digitalized programs—to assist individuals and teams in reframing these tough, disorienting situations.

One such example comes from the work of John Boyd, a prominent military strategist who served as an F-86 pilot during the Korean War. During his tour in Korea, he observed that the American pilots kept winning in air combat despite flying F-86 jets that were vastly inferior in comparison to the Russian MiG-15s that the Korean pilots were flying. The difference that gave Americans the advantage was that they had much greater cockpit visibility, allowing pilots to see out of the cockpit in all directions so that they could orient themselves more quickly and effectively than their opponents. Based on this observation, Boyd created the OODA loop: Observe, Orient, Decide, Act, and then repeat. The more quickly a pilot could repeat the loop, the more nimbly that pilot could fly. His survival depended on it! This is how the American pilots were gaining the advantage, by compressing their loops using superior observation and orientation.

Boyd extrapolated the model of the OODA loop to organizations, business, and government. Silicon Valley entrepreneurs have adopted the model as a mantra, working in OODA loops that might last days or weeks rather than seconds. However long the loops last, any method a company can find for compressing learning cycles gives that company a major competitive edge. It's a great example—just one of numerous examples of a distilled and templated model adapted to provide a roadmap for successful competitive advantage in a hostile or tumultuous environment. If you knew you could increase your competitive edge, wouldn't you reframe your thinking? And if you knew that there was a roadmap out there to help you with the reframe, wouldn't you give it a try?

> *If you knew you could increase your competitive edge, wouldn't you reframe your thinking?*

The Reframe Roadmap

Robert Lang's story illustrates the quintessential Reframe Roadmap. Once he *reoriented* and *redefined* the problem in other industries as a folding problem, it naturally followed that his colleagues *redirected* their strategies, tactics, and resources to use his origami programs to solve their newly reframed situation. Lang's reframe was complex, but the steps of the Reframe Roadmap are relatively simple. The one common theme of the Reframe Roadmap is that it's a comprehensive approach—meaning that all the steps have to be taken. From studying dozens of reframe case studies like Robert Lang, as well as personally interviewing dozens of others, it is my belief that if any of the critical reframing steps are skipped, the potential power of the reframe won't be achieved.

THE REFRAME ROADMAP:

1. Reorient   2. Redefine   3. Redirect

REORIENT

Reorienting is the narrative part of the reframe, in that it could almost be described as rewriting or restorying. Reorienting involves discovering or arriving at a new perspective, often a theme or approach that emerges from outside one's own discipline or industry, or from some idea or meme existing on the fringe of that industry or endeavor. That fresh perspective helps with understanding the endeavor, discipline, or industry differently and reorienting the narrative from that different point of view. This step encompasses Robert Lang's profound insight that, "Almost all innovation happens by making connections between fields that other people don't recognize." Decades before Lang, Arthur Koestler, in his book, *The Act of Creation*, coined the term "bisociation," which explains how any act of creation is more than a simple association of ideas but instead a "bisociation" of seemingly incompatible frames of thought—"a blending of elements drawn from two previously unrelated matrices of thought into a new matrix of meaning, by way of a process involving comparison, abstraction and categorization, analogies and metaphors."[29] Koestler writes that, "all decisive events in the history of scientific thought can be described in terms of mental cross-fertilization between different disciplines." The renowned Harvard Business School professor and author, Clayton Christensen, who coined and developed the concept of "disruptive innovation"—which has been called one of the most influential business ideas of our time—has a related commentary that supports the critical importance of this first step of the Reframe Roadmap. As I previously quoted and am quite purposefully restating, Professor Christensen puts it this way, "When the business world encounters an intractable management problem, it's a sign that there isn't yet a satisfactory theory for what's causing the problem, and under what circumstances it can be overcome."

There are numerous approaches to stimulating and structuring the reorient step of the process. One set of approaches I've encountered comes from Steven Johnson, a respected science writer, brilliant storyteller, and author of numerous books. In his 2010 *New York Times* bestseller, *Where Good Ideas Come From: The Natural History of Innovation*, he describes six patterns or environments that facilitate innovative and reorienting thinking. These include more well-known approaches like "the adjacent possible," "liquid networks," and "errors," and include other approaches he introduces such as "serendipity," "exaptation," and "platforms."

Another set of approaches comes from the work of Dr. Gary Klein, a psychologist known for his pioneering research and writings in naturalistic decision-making. Klein spent years observing and documenting how people made good decisions in real-life situations, not in laboratory settings. In his 2013 book, *Seeing What Others Don't: The Remarkable Ways We Gain Insights*, he, similarly to Steven Johnson, provides us with an understanding of the contexts that are conducive to reframing one's thinking in order to enable successful and often life-saving actions. Dr. Klein outlines three "channels"—what he calls the "The Triple Path Model"—that suggest the different routes we can take to achieving new insights and orientations. These channels are: (1) the "Contradiction Path"—recognizing and appreciating inconsistencies and using weak, divergent anchors to rebuild a story; (2) the "Connection Path"—using curiosity to recognize coincidences and spot potential implications and applications, the activity being to add a new anchor from which to rebuild a story; and (3) the "Creative Desperation Path"—which requires discarding a weak but prevalent and widely accepted anchor concept in order to escape an impasse. More than one path can be used simultaneously to create a new insight; and they all lead to a shift in how we understand and how we act, see, feel and desire. Dr. Klein also describes the real-life challenges and tensions that inhibit reorienting insights—circumstances that we face daily in our lives, in our work, and in our organizations.

A third set of approaches to stimulating reframes comes from Jeremy Gutsche in his 2015 book *Better and Faster: The Proven Path to Unstoppable Ideas*. Gutsche draws on case studies from hundreds of entrepreneurs and innovators and provides six patterns and dozens of specific tactics that increase the opportunity for reframing to occur. In fact, I first discovered the Robert Lang story through reading Gutsche's book. The patterns he and his research team have distilled include concepts such as "convergence," "divergence," "cyclicality," "redirection," "reduction," and "acceleration." I particularly appreciate the overarching "hunter versus farmer" metaphor Gutsche introduces, in which he contrasts the "farmer traps" of complacency, repetition, and protectiveness, with the "hunter instincts" of being insatiable, staying curious, and being willing to destroy.

These are just three illustrative examples I've drawn from a base of dozens of authors, innovators, entrepreneurs, scientists, strategists, and business analysts. There are a number of common principles and methods that these and numerous other reframe approaches and methodologies share. Over time, I've learned to recognize the convergent principles in this literature—in the art and applied science of reframing and reorienting. I will freely admit to you that I find it very comforting to continuously discover that multiple experts from disparate disciplines all seem to converge on a number of fundamental principles and methodologies. I also find it comforting that there is scientific rigor behind the art of reframing and reorienting.

This first step of the Reframe Roadmap—reorient—is beyond essential. However, my observation is that it's the one step that is almost always overlooked. We won't go into the many explanations for this that I've discovered in my readings and from years of personal experience. The problem is this: while you may make improvements within the existing framework of your industry and discipline, you will fall short of the transcendent, transformative solutions that will be required

There is scientific rigor behind the art of reframing and reorienting.

to move you beyond the limitations of that framework. And, in healthcare, the predominant "copy and paste" or "borrow and steal" approach will only advance us up to a point. Now, I have no problem with "borrowing and stealing" or "copying and pasting" good ideas and successful implementations. That's not the issue. My point is that if we all continue to do that—the so-called "wisdom of the crowd"—will greatly limit how fast and how far we advance our progress and performance. This large, collective "group think" will create more of a constraint than a shared and generative enablement.

REDEFINE

Redefining will likely follow organically on the heels of reorienting. After formulating a new perspective, you are likely to begin seeing the problems and challenges you're facing quite differently. They literally will not be the same problems they were before. In fact, they can't be. In one sense, the purpose of reorientation is to substitute one set of problems for another completely different set of problems. And because you're solving for a different problem set, you'll need to either find or create different tools, approaches, and techniques. By focusing on a new problem set and using new problem-solving tools, you'll almost certainly come up with a whole new set of solutions, as well as new metrics of success. Again, this is a critical step in the reframe process, and one that all too often gets overlooked, sidestepped, and shortchanged. It reminds me of the apocryphal comment attributed to Albert Einstein—the one in which he stated that if he was given an hour to find the solution to save the universe, he would spend fifty-nine minutes defining the problem and only one minute coming up with the solution. We'll spend more than a minute on this insight in the redesign section of this book, so I'll leave it at that for now.

REDIRECT

The first two steps of the Reframe Roadmap are typically the domains of boards, CEOs, and senior leadership teams, as well as perhaps innovation teams and R&D divisions. I'm not saying that those steps should be limited to those folks; but that's my observation—and even then, the consistent application of these first two steps are often limited to the most progressive, innovative, and entrepreneurial organizations. Unfortunately, even under the best of circumstances, organizational leaders and operational managers often neglect the crucial third step of the Reframe Roadmap—redirecting strategies, tactics, and resources. This step does require and demonstrate more sustained commitment, and therefore more risk than the first two steps of reorienting and redefining. This is the "taking action" part of the roadmap. It is also the part that leads to results. Without it, potential reframes get stuck in what I would label, "reframe purgatory." That is, they wallow in that twilight zone of "pilots" and "projects." I have observed that this is a sticking point for many organizations: not recognizing the importance of this strategic and tactical cascade of follow-through. It also often reflects, in my experience, a deeper divide between the most senior leadership and the mid-management of an organization, and represents a potential source of organizational distrust—a dissonance between espoused values and observed values.

A Life-Saving Reframe

What is most hopeful and empowering about the Reframe Roadmap is that it directly addresses an existential imperative for healthcare professionals. It speaks to the core meaning and purpose of our intellectual capabilities and our emotional energy—the talents and skills that are embedded in our hearts, heads, and hands. It speaks to the abundant value that is currently locked up—preventing us from fully realizing, manifesting, and sharing our purpose, our plans, and our labor. The ultimate purpose of the Reframe Roadmap is to release us from the restrictive thinking, practices, and approaches that squash our highest aims, and to allow us to connect as human beings on an individual, social, and existential level in pursuit of high-quality healthcare and good health.

Reframing is not a philosophical or academic exercise; it is an approach to issues that, as thinking and spiritual beings, we face each and every day. It is a way of seeing and addressing anew very concrete issues of how we live, and quite frankly, if we survive and thrive.

> *The ultimate purpose of the Reframe Roadmap is to release us from the restrictive thinking, practices, and approaches that squash our highest aims.*

In *Man's Search for Ultimate Meaning*, Viktor Frankl chronicles the liberating and life-saving impact of the reframe in very real terms—life and death. He was writing his book on the topic of meaning when, as fate would have it, he was shipped off with millions of others to the Nazi death camps. Life in these camps was unimaginable: harsh winters, physical brutalities, starvation, torture, humiliation, and the mass extermination of millions of people.

What Frankl observed during this living nightmare was that the people who withstood the trauma were not the ones he would have expected. They were not necessarily the strongest or brightest or most talented. They were, however, the individuals who were able to create meaning even under the most miserable, painful, and dehumanizing set of circumstances. From my perspective, what he was witnessing was the awesome life-enhancing and enabling power of reframing. These individuals—the ones who could create new meaning and purpose, who were able to reframe their situation, redefine their challenges, and redirect their strategies, tactics and resources—were the ones who could increase their chances of survival. There is likely some relatedness here to Leach's principle of the 10 percent of us who are naturally capable of this sort of survival.

My purpose in sharing this story is not to draw a parallel in any way between concentration camps and healthcare, or to critique individuals who, but for the grace of God, have endured torture or abuse of any sort. My purpose is to illustrate and underscore the immense power of the reframe and to drive home the point that an existential crisis demands a reframe. Reframing is about nothing less than how we live our lives, both individually and collectively, both personally and professionally. It is about whether we will transcend our circumstances or continue to be dominated, disrupted, and defeated by them.

Beside Frankel, there are numerous historic and modern-day epic examples of how reframing and the Reframe Roadmap I've introduced you to have been applied in the arts, literature, science, industry, agriculture, technology, medical research, public health, politics and civics, business management, the military, and in countless academic disciplines. These stories illustrate the transformative power of the reframe—not in solving problems, but instead, transcending them. They also demonstrate that all the steps in the Reframe Roadmap are relevant. Instead of spending another chapter or two recounting these stories, I'll refer you to the books already mentioned in this chapter as well as to the references at the end of this book. These books, and so many others in this expansive genre, contain literally hundreds of inspiring stories—illustrative examples of what I have discerned to be demonstrations of the Reframe Roadmap.

The Shift to Reframing

The ultimate purpose of the Reframe Roadmap is to liberate value— the value locked within ourselves, our teams, our organizations, and our communities. It's important to note that the Reframe Roadmap functions at the level of the ecosystem. What I mean by this is that it not only changes what happens within organizations. It transforms what occurs between organizations—the relationship of various stakeholders in the market. In some sense, reframing is a reengineering of the ecosystem.

> *In some sense, reframing is a reengineering of the ecosystem.*

I hope I have conveyed that reframing is not something mysterious and that it's not just a curious concept. In fact, reframing is not just a concept. It's a process or series of steps. Leaders, entrepreneurs, change agents, and professionals from various enterprises reframe all the time. The problem is that there is often not enough recognition, support, sustainment, and commitment to the follow-up, to the comprehensive steps of the roadmap. I also hope that I've been able to demonstrate that reframing is not problem-solving or process optimization. It's more akin to "problem-dissolving," or perhaps, more accurately, the exchange of a new and enabling set of problems for older, less useful ones. As we'll discover in chapter 7 on "Principles of Redesign," contrary to commonly held belief, problems actually serve a great purpose. When a problem set has run its course, or the purpose is no longer being realized, a new set of problem definitions is required. The Reframe Roadmap is the process for doing that in a more reliable, replicable, and effective way. As I've told my two children, one of the pearls of wisdom I've picked up over the past few years in speaking with and observing hundreds of successful entrepreneurs and leaders is that happiness isn't the absence of problems. Happiness is discovering and working on relevant and purposeful problems that can be pursued to craft a positive, meaningful, and value-laden change in the world.

It's been said that necessity is the mother of invention. I would suggest to you that necessity is also the mother of reframing. My goal here is to take the notion of reframing out of the realm of chance or some ephemeral, elusive phenomenon, and make it resemble an environment, approach, and methodology that can be systematized, codified, operationalized, tested, iterated, and improved upon—essentially to make it a leadership tool. At the very least, I hope that more healthcare leaders will recognize and appreciate reframes for what they can do; and more to the point, what they are already doing

> *My goal here is to take the notion of reframing out of the realm of chance to make it a leadership tool.*

in healthcare—which is greatly and irreversibly disrupting it! More of that to come in the following chapters.

Reframing is a tool kit within which lie many techniques and approaches—a mix of both the art and science. My immediate purpose is to make this tool kit more accessible to a wide audience, to the folks who can recognize and avail themselves of it—the boardroom and C-suite leaders as well as executives, managers, and change agents in large and smaller corporations—so that they can systematically and reliably turn resistant problems into solutions, and elusive solutions into manifest realities with transformative, game-changing outcomes. These outcomes will certainly provide a competitive advantage and enable these leaders and influencers to thrive in the rapidly advancing and morphing healthcare marketplace. But more importantly, the outcomes will radically improve healthcare and dramatically improve the health and well-being for ourselves, our families, our communities, our corporations, our patients, and our customers.

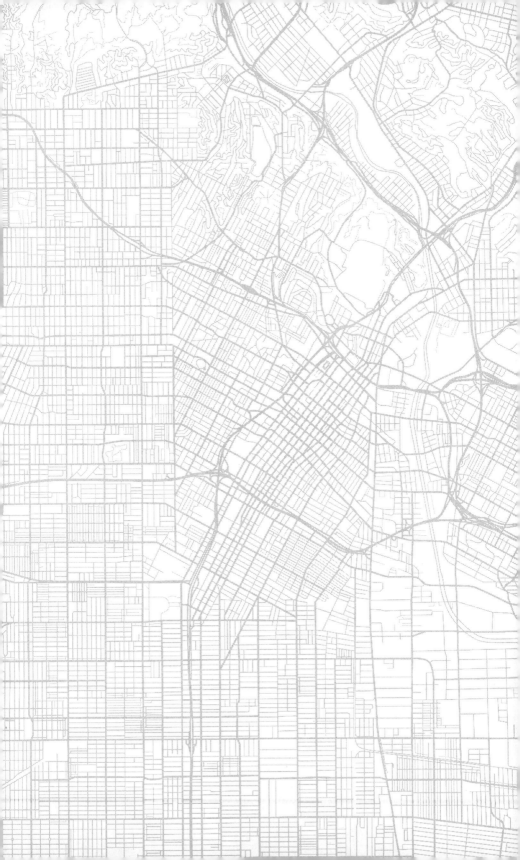

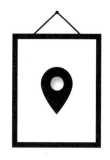

CHAPTER 3

THE MARKETING MINDSET

(A FUNDAMENTAL REFRAME TO ADDRESS THE HEALTHCARE CUSTOMER REVOLUTION)

Invention is not disruptive. Only customer adoption is disruptive.

—Jeff Bezos, founder and CEO, Amazon

In March of 2016, I was on a flight from Charlotte, North Carolina to New York City, preparing to give a presentation at a healthcare-industry conference packed with senior leaders from large hospital systems, health-insurance companies, and healthcare start-ups. The title of the talk was "What Medicine Can Learn from Marketing." Unlike just about every other talk I had given before, I had not prepared ahead of time—no PowerPoint slides, no notes, no nothing. I was going to wing it, which was completely out of character for me. I felt that I needed to do something I had never done before—to disrupt my pattern. I needed to be as raw and real as I could. I was planning to speak about something I never had brought to an audience before, and I wanted as little artifact between the idea and listeners. In the past, my presentations, at conferences like these, focused on a clinical program, project, or initiative I had led or participated in—all of them concluded with my reporting on our outstanding results and learnings. *This* talk had nothing to do with a specific program or initiative. This would be the first time I spoke exclusively about the *context* of healthcare delivery, rather than the content. This would be the first time I presented the conceptual frameworks that had been gestating in my mind for nearly a decade. I would typically get a bit nervous in the hours leading up to a talk, but surprisingly, I wasn't at all nervous this time. My belief was that context would eat content for lunch. I knew that I had been developing a very different way of looking at what was occurring and needed to occur in the healthcare world. What I needed to know was whether the healthcare world was ready for what I was about to introduce to it.

It's now nearly two years after that inaugural talk and I've continued to share and refine this approach with dozens of audiences, boards, and leadership teams. I've also now witnessed firsthand, in consulting with these teams, the power of the reframe in action. What's also been encouraging and surprising to me is that many of the groups I've spoken to have invited me back for a second and even third round. So, the healthcare world seems ready.

> The essence of marketing is to be entirely focused on the consumer.

This chapter introduces the reframe that I'm calling the *Marketing Mindset*. Why "Marketing?" Because the essence of marketing is to be entirely focused on the customer. The core of that discipline (again, both art and science) is to seek to understand others. One of the driving assumptions behind this reframe is a simple one: the healthcare system should see the people coming to it as people, not as patients—but instead as VIP customers, consumers, and clients—and focus its energies, efforts, and outcomes entirely on them. Everything I've discovered, observed, and studied over the past few decades has led me to believe that it is time for us to rid ourselves of the anachronistic conceptual frame of the "patient" and adopt a new theory of people seeking healthcare—more akin to "healthcare customers."

Critical point here: when I talk about or use the term "marketing," I'm not talking about public relations, media relations, advertising, or sales. I'm not talking about billboards, commercials, radio spots, or even social-media marketing. I'm talking about the underlying fundamental principles of marketing in their most up-to-date and evolved state. I believe that by adopting and leveraging what I'm labelling as the Marketing Mindset, we can reorient healthcare through the broad lens of marketing to fundamentally and radically improve how consumers purchase, utilize, experience, and benefit from healthcare. In other words, what I'm talking about is adopting and adapting the essence of marketing—the principles, techniques, and technologies that draw our attention to deep human needs and desires.

Humanizing Healthcare

I spent the first dozen years of my career as an academic teaching physician. My academic focus was on trying to understand why patients were not heard and understood as people, and coming up with ways to improve the patient situation. My work centered on enhancing the ability of physicians, nurses, and other providers to demonstrate empathy for their patients. While most of my colleagues and contemporaries were focused on the technological aspects of care, it seemed to me that the humanistic aspects were lagging. I also observed very early on in my career that, in the rapidly evolving industrial complex of healthcare delivery, the humanistic treatment of healthcare providers was also lagging.

I made it my career goal to create the environment patients needed to voice their perspectives—not just about the clinical, physical, and functional issues at hand, but also about the emotional, relational, and social aspects of well-being that are often abandoned in the name of efficiency, productivity, and clinical effectiveness. I was in the healing profession, and I couldn't understand how we could ignore the fact that illness and disease weren't isolated phenomena but contextual ones. Both from a causative and curative perspective, people's illnesses were part of their lives, their entire lives, and not just isolated or limited to their physical anatomy and physiology. To put it plainly, it seemed to me that patients were more than their condition or disease. But the systemic approach we took in healthcare didn't recognize, reward, or provide a reliable and replicable roadmap for responding to that seemingly obvious and important understanding.

Marketing 101

I realized early on in my academic career that I wasn't going to change the world in the way I had hoped for—by sitting in an exam room taking care of patients or by teaching internal-medicine residents. I found the practice of medicine to be interesting, challenging and rewarding on many levels. I also loved my patients and was devoted to them; but this wasn't the primary path I needed to pursue in order to transform healthcare delivery. I had already begun consulting to leadership teams in hospital systems across the country, and I began to think that moving into a consulting position would allow me to create more leverage for humanizing healthcare. However, one thing I noticed in my organizational consulting engagements was that the administrative leaders and I were not speaking the same language. They were using a different conceptual framework from the one I had been trained in. Their language was that of management, finance, accounting, and clinical operations. I knew that if I was to make the transition into being a valuable healthcare consultant or advisor, I would need to understand those conceptual frames and have some facility in those disciplines. I didn't have a background in business or health management at the time, but I knew that I had to augment my own framework if I was going to enact the changes that I believed healthcare so desperately needed.

So, I returned to grad school at the Harvard School of Public Health for a master's program in healthcare management, targeted at mid-career physician-executives. In the second year of that program, I took a Marketing 101 course, and it was a game changer. I recall sitting in those marketing classes, month after month, in the stadium-like lecture halls typical of business schools. I had this bizarre but thrilling realization about the core elements of the discipline of marketing. I recall the sensation of buzzing with enthusiasm as the highly-experienced instructor—Linda MacCracken—shared the concepts and the business case studies. I couldn't take notes fast enough nor write down the ideas that were being spawned in my mind. At times, I would look to my left and right, at my colleagues sitting next to me. They did not seem to resonate with or perceive what I was discovering. The theories, the fundamental elements, the tools and techniques of marketing—these were all much more sophisticated and far better ways of doing what I had been attempting to do my entire career—to humanize healthcare! Everyone else around me was understanding the application of marketing as a way to promote the healthcare business—to advertise hospitals and provider groups; but I saw it as a way to actually deliver healthcare!

> Marketing could be used not to sell healthcare, but to do healthcare!

Marketing could be used not to sell healthcare, but to do healthcare! I thought to myself, "If we could transpose some of those concepts onto healthcare delivery, it would vastly improve our ability to take care of people, to enhance their experience of care, and to achieve the health outcomes we were espousing."

The "Marketing Mindset" emerged for me in exactly the way that Albert Einstein, Robert Lang, Arthur Koestler and numerous others have described—that innovations or solutions to dilemmas come from outside of the mindset in which they arose. Referencing Gary Klein's model, I was experiencing a combination of the "Connection" and "Creative Desperation" pathways to new insight—discarding old anchors and finding new ones. Or, what Art Koestler termed, "bisociation"—bringing disparate and seemingly incompatible schools of thought together. For me, Marketing 101 was my "Steve Jobs moment," the moment when I knew that converting marketing into a mindset for approaching healthcare delivery could radically change healthcare delivery and the industry itself.

One side note: The field of marketing continues to evolve, and I've continued to learn and borrow from it and other fields, including approaches taken from content marketing, predictive analytics, customer relationship management, pre- and post-marketing, digital marketing, social media, customer journey mapping, human centered design, empathy or emotion mapping, the lean start-up methodology, and so on. My purpose here is not to dive into or explain all these topics. The concepts and approaches derived from these disciplines, however, are woven throughout the course of this book.

Over the course of my thirteen-year experience learning about marketing and consumerism, I have adapted a simple way of understanding the basic elements which include: *identifying* who our customers are, *focusing* on segments of customers, *understanding* their specific needs and their particular journeys, *customizing* a solution that is relevant to their needs and goals, and *engaging* them in a way that creates and sustains that relevance.

THE FUNDAMENTAL CONSUMERIST MARKETING MINDSET:

1. IDENTIFY your customers
2. Focus on certain customer SEGMENTS
3. UNDERSTAND their specific needs/journey
4. Create CUSTOMIZED, RELEVANT SOLUTIONS that meet THEIR needs
5. ENGAGE them so needs and solutions are CONNECTED and SUSTAINED

What is fascinating to me about these basic marketing steps is that they are consistent with what I had taught my internal-medicine residents-in-training years ago. I taught them to understand their patients and their patients' specific needs; to adapt the clinical medicine they had learned and apply it to each unique patient; and then to engage the patient in an iterative treatment plan. The difference for me, however, is that the Marketing Mindset puts patient-centered care on steroids. Instead of the seat-of-the-pants psychoso-cial training most of us in healthcare receive, the field of marketing brings to bear decades of science, advanced technologies and analytics, and sophisticated, quantifiable techniques. From my perspective, providers have, in many ways, been using these tools; but now we can incorporate a field and a discipline that provides us with a detailed framework of the individual patient as a thinking, feeling, social, cultural, and existential being. The Marketing Mindset provides healthcare with the science and art to explore and understand people. As a result, it can help fill a profound gap in our ability to fulfill our mission as a healing and health-care profession.

> *The Marketing Mindset provides healthcare with the science and art to explore and understand people. As a result, it can help fill a profound gap in our ability to fulfill our mission as a healing and healthcare profession.*

From Identifying to Engaging your Customer

I'd like to jump right into an articulation of these basic elements of marketing I listed in The Fundamental Consumerist Marketing Mindset. One of the first steps in a marketing approach is to identify your customer. A few starter questions to ask include:

- For whom are you attempting to create value?

- Who are your customers, and what do they want or need?

- What do you know about their lives and how are you exploring that?

- What is their experience of solving specific problems in their lives?

- How have you explored the heterogeneity of your customers' needs?

The next step is to focus on certain segments of customers, and that's closely tied to the third point above: understanding your customers' needs and journeys. The idea of segmentation is based on the understanding that you can't be all things for all people, all the time; and that if you try to do that, you'll likely end up being nothing special for anyone most of the time. Segmentation is the understanding that while it's challenging and often impractical to individualize products or services for every single person, you can customize by segmenting groups or categories of people, needs, and situational contexts. Segmentation can be done in lots of ways: by gender, age, or income; by social demographics; by life stage or situation; or by a specific condition or set of needs. The point is that segmentation allows you to better understand a problem or need that is shared by a sub-segment of a population and therefore allows you to create a more customized solution for that need and for that segment. It's a way to create greater understanding of your customers and to create greater value for them. But even within segments of the population, it's also imperative to understand that each customer does have more specific needs. Another question to consider: if you believe you already know what your customers want, how exactly do you know that? How have you confirmed your knowledge? Have you asked them directly (which carries its own pitfalls)? Have you learned about their past behaviors and the factors that weigh heavily in their decision making? Have you learned how they make their decisions and who makes those decisions? Have you discovered their influencers? What the customer wants may not be immediately apparent; in fact, even within customer segments, it often isn't obvious at first blush.

The fourth step in this simplified model is to rapidly create a customized solution to meet a customer's real needs and test that prototype; and a fifth step is to connect your solution to that need with the surrounding para-products. In other words, it's not simply enough to provide customers with a tool. You must also engage customers and maintain relevance by providing them ways to be active in their own care. That's not an easy feat; but the technologies now available to develop and continuously personalize solutions and enhance engagement are vast and very much available to us in healthcare. This isn't a reinvention of the wheel. The tools exist; we just need to use them.

Again, when you pause to think about it, the distilled principles of the Marketing Mindset parallel the distilled basis of medical care. Consider this: the first step in treating a patient is diagnosis—identifying what the problem is. The second step is to create a customized treatment plan, to figure out what makes this patient unique and how to adapt what we know from the evidence-based literature and our training to treat this patient—the singular person in front of you. The third step for a responsible medical professional is to ensure that patients follow through with the treatment plan, that they connect

> *The ability to connect the client with the solution—to create relevance and engagement—is a critically important part of providing good medical care.*

to the solution. It's not sufficient to merely dispense the prescription or make the referral. I often hear providers say that they can't make their patients follow through. No, they can't, but our collective job is to educate, influence, and engage patients so that they have the best chance of becoming active participants in their own care. Part of our job, in a sense, is marketing medicine or healthcare. The patient given an antibiotic prescription for pneumonia who does not fill that script and take the medication is going to end up sicker. This can lead not only to bad outcomes but also to greatly increased costs of care. So, the ability to connect the client with the solution—to create relevance and engagement—is a critically important part of providing good medical care.

Demand-Side Thinking—A "Consumer-Only" Approach

As an industry, healthcare is largely focused on its internal stakeholders. Whenever we engage in internal tactical or operational discussions, one of the underlying and unspoken principles is an "all-stakeholder" approach—to guarantee that providers, administrators, staff and everyone else feels good about any new initiative, process, program, or direction. At worst, it can devolve into mostly making sure that we meet the needs of the people in the room rather than meeting the needs of our patients. Is it convenient for us? Is it a priority for us? How does it impact our performance metrics? How does it affect our workflow and compensation? It's what I now refer to as a "consumer-also" approach, rather than a "consumer-centric" or "consumer-only" approach. When you stop to think about it, it seems a bit backwards—starting with us first, rather than starting with the consumer. That internal focus is what I've heard described as "supply-side thinking" versus "demand-side thinking."

As I've sat in meetings over the years, I've wondered to myself:

"Would software engineers in Silicon Valley be asked if a new software program met their needs? Would managers or distributors or developers in a large retail chain be asked if a new product line or service met their needs?"

Of course not! It's ludicrous. Every successful retailer understands that it's a consumer-only mindset and approach that determines your ability to create value and thrive in the market. In fact, it's often inconvenient and untimely to make customer-driven change, but it's what competitive retailers must do if they are to remain relevant. In full disclosure, I had never heard of the phrase "customer-only" until I spoke with someone outside of the healthcare industry—Marcus Osborne, the VP of health and wellness products and services at Walmart.[30] We'll return to this concept again. And as Marcus and many others will attest, the supply-side thinking trap is not limited to healthcare. As Jeremy Gutsche, CEO of trendhunters.com eloquently states, "It's funny how you can become such an expert that you lose touch with how your customers think… One of the things I learned along the way is that sometimes you have to unlearn what you think is great. Then you can open yourself up to what your customer is really thinking."[31]

Needless to say, we must abide by regulatory and legal requirements; and in healthcare, there are numerous quality and safety requirements. We must also understand that what we design and organize can't be something that puts undue pressure on providers and staff. It's got to be doable and sustainable. I'm not questioning any of those functional constraints. But I am challenging the systemic notion that a primary directive should be to discover from all internal stakeholders whether or not a change or redesign meets their needs, as opposed to the primary directive being meeting the needs of our customers. Think about those earlier questions: Who is the consumer or customer? It's not the doctor, administrator, the hospital, or the payer; but I've heard many healthcare leaders speak as if these constituents were their primary customer base. Fortunately, I'm observing less and less of this as the market evolves into a more competitive and consumerist one.

On the other hand, there is good reason and good evidence for treating your teammates and colleagues as internal VIP customers. I am a vocal proponent of that approach to leadership, management, teamwork, and collegiality. I have learned and discovered that if you treat your people well, that will enable them to treat their customers well. For me, it boils down to an issue of integrity and trust. But, this can't be at the expense of understanding and serving your customers, and providing the best possible experience, care and outcomes. The take-home point is that we have to shift from a "customer-also" mindset and adopt the "customer-only"

> *We have to shift from a "customer-also" mindset and adopt the "customer-only" mindset.*

mindset if we are going to participate in, contribute to, and thrive in the predominant Marketing Mindset healthcare reframe.

Supply-side thinking is necessary and cannot be ignored. We need to focus on the internal workings of our business, for sure. But, it's most definitely not enough for meeting the needs of healthcare customers. As we look back over the past few decades, one can observe that our predominant supply-side thinking approach has kept our healthcare system in largely the same state. And as long as we remain in that mindset, we will never transform healthcare.

Process improvement and efficiency experts would inform us that even incremental value-laden changes do not come from supply-side thinking. Meaningful value-laden change of any significance requires a demand-side orientation.

Demand-side thinking requires an external focus. It's a focus on what the customers' problems are, what "good" would look like from their perspective, and what obstacles and challenges are getting in the way of them achieving the results and outcomes they desire. Demand-side orientation requires the supplier to be open to shifting, changing, and pivoting in order to meet the needs of the customer. This can be challenging to organizations, since most are wired to keep the trains running on the track and on time. But, if the healthcare industry were to fully embrace a continuous customer-only, demand-side approach, it could literally transform healthcare delivery and health outcomes.

If the healthcare industry were to fully embrace a continuous customer-only, demand-side approach, it could literally transform healthcare delivery and health outcomes.

The following questions provide an introductory guide as to whether you and your organization are engaged predominantly in demand-side or supply-side thinking. As you read these questions, think about yourself, your teams, your providers, managers, and staff. What type of questions are you asking and responding to? Think about your patient experience surveys. What questions are they asking and what thinking does that represent? I suspect that once you begin to deploy these questions, you'll start generating even more specific and relevant questions.

QUESTIONS THAT SUGGEST A PREDOMINANTLY SUPPLY-SIDE, CUSTOMER-ALSO PERSPECTIVE:

- How well do you (the customer) know me/us?

- How well do I/we perform?

- How satisfied are you (the customer) with me/us?

- How do I make you (the customer) understand me/us better?

- How do I make you (the customer) understand my/our decision-making process and my perspectives?

- How do I make you (the customer) understand my/our challenges and obstacles?

- How do I make you (the customer) understand what's inside my/our head?

- How do I create or unleash value for me/us?

- How do I inform and convince you (the customer) of how good I am/we are?

QUESTIONS THAT SUGGEST A PREDOMINANTLY DEMAND-SIDE OR CUSTOMER-ONLY PERSPECTIVE:

- How well do I/we know you (the customer)?

- How do I/we understand you (the customer) better?

- How well do I/we understand your needs and concerns, problems, hopes, and desires?

- How well do I/we understand your challenges and obstacles to obtaining what you desire/need?
- How well am I/are we meeting your needs?
- How do I/we understand and engage you (the customer) better?
- How do I/we understand your decision-making process and your perspective?
- How do I/we understand what's inside your head and heart?
- How well are you (the customer) performing?
- How do I/we understand and enhance your potential?
- How do I/we create, enable or unleash value for you (the customer)?
- How do I/we show you how good you are and how good you might become?

Examples of *Consumer-Only* versus *Consumer-Also* Approaches

Lowes is one of the best examples of a demand-side oriented business. I first heard about this from a colleague, Ann Somers-Hogg. Lowe's sells tools and supplies to assist people in jobs around the house and yard. They are experts in the tools and supplies business. One way to market themselves would be to tout the quality or the expanse of their offerings. Similar stores have gone the route of emphasizing what they offer by promoting the quality and/or selection of their tools. No matter how true those claims about quality may be, their focus, thinking, and perspective is internal. It is necessary to provide high-quality supplies; but doing so is not sufficient for becoming a successful and beloved business.

Let's look at how Lowe's markets itself to its customers. First, Lowe's has reframed itself as a "home-improvement warehouse," as opposed to a "tool and supply warehouse." Instead of promoting themselves for what they sell or do, they are recognizing and promoting the need and solution that the customer is looking for. Lowe's also takes a demand-side approach with their tagline: "Love where you live." With this statement, they are—I would add, brilliantly so—making explicit their understanding of the customer's ultimate goal. They have taken a demand-side perspective and recognized both the challenge and the goal for the customer. Granted, a business cannot just market itself as these things without also showing and being truthful about what they market. But Lowe's does that as well. From a Reframe Roadmap perspective, Lowes is redefining and reorganizing itself within a demand-side orientation.

In contrast to Lowe's success, the demise of the Kodak company is a classic example of the disastrous consequences of maintaining a predominantly "supply-side" orientation. It's a highly instructive case study that has profound implications for healthcare today. Like many others, I had been under the impression that Kodak's downfall, following decades of profound success and dominance in the photography market, was the result of myopic leadership. I had assumed that, although Kodak had developed the digital camera back

> *The demise of the Kodak company is a classic example of the disastrous consequences of maintaining a predominantly "supply-side" orientation.*

in 1975, it ultimately ignored that advance and fell far behind its competitors. I recently learned that this is not the true story. Although Kodak was a little late to the game, it made huge investments in digital technologies and huge strategic decisions to shut down film factories and lay off tens of thousands of film-factory workers. In fact, by 2005, Kodak was number one in digital-camera sales in the US and number three in digital-camera sales globally! Kodak had developed over one-thousand patents related to digital image capture and received billions of dollars in licensing fees, including patent fees received from competitors such as Samsung and LG. They invested and reinvested heavily in critical intellectual digital technologies.[32]

So, if they weren't the disruptive-innovation luddites that many of us suspected they were, what went wrong? The problem was that they focused on what they wanted, and not what the evolving customers and emerging market wanted. As digital technologies advanced with greater phone- and computer-screen image resolutions and greater photo memory capacity, customers were increasingly wanting to see and store their photos on phones, laptops and desktop computers. Kodak, however, was focused internally, and saw digital as a way to feed its high-margin printing-service line. They assumed that as digital photography's market presence increased, the need and demand for digital printing would increase. So, they were banking on that and investing hugely in their high-margin printer ink and photo-paper division. But that's not what their customer base wanted or needed. Because they had a predominant supply-side orientation, their leadership missed the game-changing shift that was taking place around them. They went through a slow, painful, and preventable demise, which ended in their filing for bankruptcy in 2012; only a few short years after they had dominated the market, and despite their investment and dominance in the advancing digital technologic era. That's a harsh but important lesson in the dangers of supply-side thinking; and it's particularly chilling as we observe some of the strategies and tactics of today's legacy healthcare systems. Another corollary lesson here for healthcare leaders is that the mere adoption of digital and other advancing technologies is not, in and of itself, a safeguard approach to competitive survival in the digital age. A demand-side, customer-only Marketing Mindset is, however, the safeguard to remaining relevant and thriving.

A couple of more examples—this time from within the healthcare system—will help us further understand the difference between demand-side and supply-side thinking. The highways of many cities in this country are lined with billboards advertising local hospitals and medical centers. Think about how those billboards present healthcare and how it's being promoted. How many of those billboards tout hospitals by advertising the best surgeons or the best doctors or, more specifically, the best orthopedists or best neurosurgeons? How many of them list their awards and recognitions, almost like a resume? How many times have you seen the slogan "We are #1 in …?"

Because we've become so numb to these advertisements, the billboards seem normal, even sensible. No question, the technical expertise of individuals and teams within a hospital system or provider group is critically important. And I'm not even suggesting that these billboards don't have an impact. When your local competitor is touting these claims, it's more of a defensive marketing strategy to toot your own horn. But, when we put our demand-side, customer-only hat on, we can begin to appreciate how these messages are skewed toward the industry and aren't very much about the customers or consumers. For starters, what does your being "number 1" or being the "best" actually mean in terms of my needs and my outcomes as a patient? I'm not being daft, and I do understand the intended implications of those statements. But the point is that this is still about you and not about me, as a customer, consumer, and client. What I want to know is, "What problems can you solve for me, as a customer, and how well can you solve them?" Recall the contrasting Lowe's demand-side orientation and customer-only tag line. What we've been selling in healthcare is a story about ourselves—an internally oriented, supply-side story. When I observe the supply-side orientation in healthcare, I see an immense opportunity for new consumer-only competitors to enter and take over.

At this point, I actually find it embarrassing when I witness how focused healthcare can be on itself instead of on its customers. The slippery slope is that it can become predominantly about our "our people, our expertise, our technology, our internal strategies and tactics." But the reality is that customers are focused on their problems, their needs, their desires, their solutions, and their stories. Kodak's leadership didn't get it, but Kaiser Permanente's does.

A great example of demand-side orientation in healthcare is Kaiser Permanente, or KP, a large healthcare system (provider group and insurance company) based in California. I was struck by KP's billboards years ago, even before I understood or appreciated the concept of demand-side versus supply-side thinking. KP has a one-word tagline—"Thrive"—and all their billboards present some variation on this theme. It's powerfully moving, inviting, and engaging.

What is the difference in this approach from the healthcare billboards we usually see? KP isn't telling its customer base that they've got the best doctors or the most doctors, the most recognitions, or the best robots or emergency rooms. They do have top-notch, industry-leading quality and performance metrics, but they don't lead with that. The focus is not on themselves, but on you, the healthcare customer. The story they tell is not their story. It's your story. The subtext here (in my words) is, "We can solve your problem. We can help you not only survive but actually thrive and live a better, healthier, and happier life. We'll take care of all your healthcare needs, so you can focus on living an active, robust, energetic, relationship-filled, happy, and meaningful life." And, I suspect that KP will not be the only one to adopt this approach in the emerging hypercompetitive market. With the retail-giants' entry into healthcare—corporations like Amazon, Google, Apple, Walmart, Walgreens, CVS, and so on; you can be assured they're not going to take a "customer-also" approach, but will instead adopt a demand-side, customer-only orientation, similar to KP's. While the legacy healthcare system has been distracted, spending time and energy focused on trying to keep their internal stakeholders happy and optimizing internal processes, these emerging new-entrant giants will be primarily focused on understanding, serving, and meeting our healthcare customers' needs.

Now, I don't want you to think that demand-side thinking is satisfied by a handful of well-designed advertisements. It's not achieved by leadership declaring it so, adding some words to your organization's strategic plan, launching a consumer initiative, or deploying some digital technologies. It's a discipline, and it requires disciplined practitioners. It's certainly not our default mindset in healthcare,

> *While the legacy healthcare system has been distracted ... these emerging new-entrant giants will be primarily focused on understanding, serving and meeting our healthcare customers' needs.*

although I've been seeing an increasing movement toward it, which is a hopeful sign. But what I'm talking about is adopting this as the primary way of thinking and performing, in all aspects of healthcare delivery. Like any organizational or cultural behavior change, it requires a roadmap—a plan of implementation, resourcing, tracking, and adjusting. This is particularly true when, as in healthcare today, the old behavior is so ingrained and so habitual. One quick rule of thumb here, before we dive into the details: if it feels uncomfortable, awkward and painful, chances are that you're on the right track. If it feels comfortable, chances are that you've slipped back into supply-side thinking. Demand-side thinking is, by its nature, disorienting and reorienting. It will require retraining, observation, and ongoing coaching. It will require the follow-up steps of redesigning and reorganizing. It will require a Marketing Mindset.

The Marketing Mindset and Your Value Proposition

Demand-side thinking should lead healthcare professionals to think about their value propositions differently. We need to realize that our value proposition is not what we want or what we want to do. It's the customers who ultimately define value. Now, we may want to help shape that value, but we are not the ones who initially get to define it. The value proposition is a co-creation between the customer and the supplier. Ultimately, the highly personal, emotional, and social needs of healthcare customers are the real drivers behind our value proposition. The Marketing Mindset helps us realize and proactively respond to the basic human needs expressed by our customers—the need to be heard, understood, and attended to on a physical, emotional, relational, and existential level. So far, I've identified the fundamental elements of marketing that can be used to guide how you develop your products and services for your customers, and how you interact with consumers. If you'll recall, the elements of this approach were to identify who your customers are, focus on a specific segment, understand their specific needs and journey, customize solutions relevant to this customer segment's needs and goals, and engage these customers in their own care. What I want to introduce to you now are the four steps of Marketing Mindset that fit within the Reframe Roadmap outlined in chapter 2. These four steps are critical and essential for any seriously attempted reframe within healthcare organizations and the overall healthcare system.

THE STEPS OF THE MARKETING MINDSET ARE:

1. **Rebrand**
2. **Redesign**
3. **Results**
4. **Reorganize**

These basic elements of the Marketing Mindset reframe are synergistic with the Reframe Roadmap. When you combine and insert the Marketing Mindset into the Reframe Roadmap it turns out that there are actually seven steps in the model:

1.   Reorient—by discovering and adopting a new perspective;

2.   Redefine—the problem from within that new orientation;

3.   Rebrand—using a new value proposition derived from your reorienting and redefining;

4.   Redesign—from the new perspective and proposition and with the new outcome(s) in mind;

5.   Results—identify the new outcomes and new metrics, with the end-goal in mind which is to deliver demand-side, customer-only value;

6.   Reorganize—based on all of the previous steps, the current structure is likely suboptimal in supporting the reoriented rebrand, facilitating the redesign, and delivering on the new value proposition and results. This will also require you to...

7.   Redirect—your strategies, tactics, and resources—a critical stop demonstrating your integrity, your true support, follow-up, and actual commitment to the reframe.

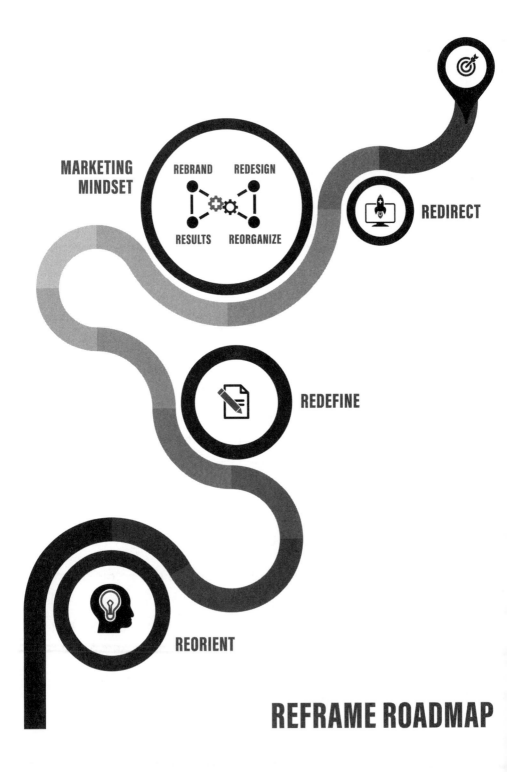

MARKETING MINDSET

REBRAND   REDESIGN

RESULTS   REORGANIZE

REDIRECT

REDEFINE

REORIENT

REFRAME ROADMAP

The Healthcare-Customer Revolution

Are you ready to learn how to create disruptive positive change in healthcare? If so, welcome to the healthcare-customer revolution where "customer-centered care is the new patient-centered care." I realize that this is not yet a popular perspective, particularly among providers; and it may draw quite a bit of concern and ire. So, I'm asking you to keep an open mind as we explore the differences as I see them. I believe that we're trying to get to the same place and the same outcome. What I'm suggesting is a different path, and a different language.

> *Customer-centered care is the new patient-centered care.*

Over the past couple of years, I've been formulating and sharing my understanding that customer-oriented care is highly empathetic and ethical care—perhaps even more-so than our current patient-centered care model. It's been said that "language is reality." We sometimes need to change our language and our narrative in order to change our reality. From my perspective, the language of consumerism—of patients as consumers, customers, and clients—is a narrative that will enable us to focus on and deliver much greater respect, dignity, value, and outcomes. In order to make the great leap to a Marketing Mindset, I strongly suspect that we will need to change our language, our narrative and our thinking from caring for "patients" to serving "healthcare customers." I will admit that I still struggle with some of the terminology—how to use and distinguish among the words—customer, consumer, client—for example. I have some thoughts about this, but the overriding issue and more challenging one is the conversion from patient to a customer/consumer mindset. For the sake of simplicity and consistency, I'll just go with the term "customer" for now.

Look at the lists below and compare the "legacy patient" framework to the "healthcare customer" framework. This is just a starter list. I suspect that you can and will generate much better and more comprehensive comparisons. But the point is this: as you read through, think about which framework you would prefer for yourself, your family and your friends.

LEGACY PATIENT	HEALTHCARE CUSTOMER
Patient is passive	Customer is active and proactive
Patient is disempowered	Customer has tremendous agency
Patient waits	Customer is waited upon
Patient is acted upon	Customer is served
Patient must be "compliant" or "adherent"	Customer is engaged
Patient suffers	Customer seeks resolution
Patient must listen and adhere	Customer is listened and adhered to
Patients evokes sympathy	Customer evokes respect
Patient is object of clinical attention	Customer's problem or need is the objective
Patient has a disease	Customer has a situation, problem, need, or desire

LEGACY PATIENT	HEALTHCARE CUSTOMER
Patient is referred to by a disease or anatomic part	Customer is referred to as a person
Patient accepts whatever care is offered	Customer shops for best option
Patient does not inquire about quality, service, or outcomes	Customer expects and demands transparent information about quality, service, and outcomes
Patient does not question authority	Customer questions authority and expertise
Patient does not have a sense of outcome	Customer has clear sense of expectations and outcomes
Patient does not expect standardized service	Customer will walk away when service standardization and reliability waver

The root of the word "patient" derives from the word for "suffering." I believe that we need to shift from a focus on suffering to a focus on health, and shift from the idea of the patient (the person as the sufferer) to healthcare customer (the person seeking health and well-being). The former notion made sense in the remote past, when there was not much one could do for someone with illness except attempt to minimize their suffering. It made sense in the remote past when the focus was on mitigating the impact of disease and trauma, as opposed to optimizing health and wellness. Now, however, we work to prevent and rid disease, improve health, and optimize our overall well-being. So, my belief is that while the "patient" and "patient-centered care" concepts served a purpose in the past, they are now anachronistic, limiting, and even harmful. The reality is that the concept of "the patient" is already shifting to that of "the customer." My hope is that we embrace, support, and accelerate this change to a customer-centric mindset.

One day, about a year ago, I was working with a group of health-care-system clients and their vendor organization, which had sponsored an advisory retreat. I encouraged them to consider the differences between "patient" and "customer." I turned to the crowd and asked, "How many of you here want to be a 'patient'?" No one raised their hands. I continued, "And when you become a patient—because the vast majority of us will sooner or later end up in that role—how many of you are planning to be a patient 'patient'?" Again, not one hand went up. I went on, "How many of you are a patient person?" Again, no one raised their hands. Not one person wanted to be a patient, a patient "patient," or even identified as a patient person for that matter. Now, this was a crowd of very forward-thinking physician leaders, highly accomplished executives, and driven entrepreneurs. I wasn't surprised that no one in the room wanted to be a patient person or a patient "patient." So, then I asked, "How many of you want to be treated like a VIP healthcare customer?" Almost everyone's hand shot up. "So, here's the point," I continued. "Why do we think it's ok for others to be a patient 'patient', if we wouldn't want to be one ourselves? And, why do we think it's ok for us to be treated like VIP healthcare customers, but not our patients?" I saw nods in the crowd. It was clear that we all agreed that we needed a more humanistic, empathetic, and people-centered model. I was just advocating for a new language and a new narrative to get us there.

> I turned to the crowd and asked, "How many of you here want to be a 'patient'?" No one raised their hands.

The point I'm trying to drive home is that a customer-only Marketing Mindset approach has the potential to enable us to deliver a more humanistic and empathetic healthcare experience, and in essence, more truly patient-centered outcomes. We have, for decades, been talking about "patient-centered" care. It is the right idea with the right purpose. But, this orientation, language, and narrative is mired in the legacy objectification, decontextualization, and depersonalization of people as medical conditions or diseases. I believe that, regardless of our immediate support, the conceptual frame and narrative of the "patient" will become less and less relevant as the Marketing Mindset reframe and the emerging megatrends in healthcare transform our thinking and delivery of healthcare services and products.

Addressing Concerns About Patients as Customers

I've heard three major arguments opposing the adoption of the "healthcare customer" term and narrative. All are based, in my estimation, on a misunderstanding of consumerism and a rose-colored interpretation of our current patient-centered care deployment.

The first opposing argument is this: If we adopt a "customer-only" approach, our goals and our metrics will become focused on selling (or perhaps overselling) more products and services, instead of doing what's medically appropriate for the patient.

The second opposing argument is this: Patients often come to providers wanting or preferring a medication or treatment that is not evidence-based or clinically appropriate. Taking a consumer-only approach would place the provider in an ethical bind. The choice being either to give the customers what they want or deliver the appropriate care.

The third opposing argument is this: Healthcare does not represent typical "customer" situations. Unlike in other industries where people are generally feeling well, interested in, and even knowledgeable about a product or service, patients may very well be in a vulnerable state due to infirmity, weakness, pain, anxiety, fear, and be absent of the knowledge or information that could contribute to their decision-making. Offering healthcare is not like selling a caffè latte or providing an amusement-park-like experience.

Each of these arguments is genuine and based on valid experience. However, in my estimation, they're also based on a lack of understanding of consumerism (which is totally understandable), and perhaps a somewhat selective or idealistic interpretation of our current patient-centered care deployment. Let's address them one by one.

First Argument: Let's tackle the issue of the idealistic and selective interpretation of our current system. It's a bit like throwing stones from a glass house when we, in healthcare, talk about "selling" or "over selling" products and services. The amount of overutilization—of inappropriate, unnecessary, and avoidable services—is one of the more shameful realities of our current so-called "patient-centered" healthcare system. It would be hard to imagine that we could do much worse than we're doing now, on this account. The truth is that healthcare continues to work largely in a volume-based payment, productivity mode. Hospitals, healthcare systems, and provider groups, by and large, work to metrics of volume—more visits, more tests, more imaging studies, more referrals, more procedures, more surgeries, more medications, and more hospital beds filled. There are productivity or "volume" goals for the majority of divisions and providers within our healthcare system.

So, my first response to this objection is that we already push more and sell more clinical services than is appropriate or ethical. Patients are already experiencing this potential downside of consumerism, without any of the potential upsides or benefits. My second response, however, is to undo our assumptions about crude sales tactics, and not to equate that with consumerism. An ethical and responsible customer or consumerist approach is not about selling more. It's about providing people with what they want and even more so, what they need. It's about filling a gap or addressing a desire for an improved state.

> *An ethical and responsible customer or consumerist approach is not about selling more. It's about providing people with what they want and even more so, what they need.*

Second Argument: In speaking with consumer experts outside of healthcare, I've discovered that I didn't really understand customer service. Yes—the customer may always be right. But, it's a professional consumerist responsibility to deliver products and services within the guidelines of safety and quality. Good customer service isn't necessarily just about giving customers what they want. It's about taking good care of them. I would suggest that inappropriate treatment and overutilization isn't going to be increased by adopting a consumerist orientation. The majority of overutilization and inappropriate care in healthcare today is actually supply-side driven, not demand-side driven. It comes from us pushing, not from patients pulling. We, the collective healthcare industry, have created most of the problem. And again, just like in other industries—food, airline, energy, retail—built into healthcare consumerism would have to be quality, safety, and service standards. It's a false choice—a misunderstanding of consumerism—to paint an either/or scenario: either safe quality care or customer service. In those situations where the patient clearly wants something a provider cannot in good conscience deliver, the provider's ethical response should be the same, no matter what the overarching model—patient care or healthcare customer care.

Third Argument: It's true, healthcare does not seem to share a lot of similarities with Disneyland or Starbucks. But the consumerist approach and customer-service orientation one experiences at Disneyland or Starbucks are based on principles that apply to anyone— whether they feel well or not, whether they are ill, or in pain, or literally dying. The consumer approach is one of identifying a person's needs on multiple levels—physical, emotional, relational, and existential—creating and deploying a customized solution, and then engaging that person to create and sustain relevance. Now, clinical care and healthcare delivery is complex, the provider/patient relationship can be unique, and there are very real challenges to obtaining and providing reliable and accurate quality and cost information. A current debate on the table is whether or not healthcare consumers have the information, analytic tools, and capability to be discerning customers, and to make healthful choices. I would suggest that these factors are being addressed in the ongoing transition of healthcare into a consumerist model. It is the industry's responsibility to make it easy for customers

> *The consumer approach is one of identifying a person's needs on multiple levels—physical, emotional, relational, and existential— creating and deploying a customized solution, and then engaging that person to create and sustain relevance.*

to be discerning. The healthcare industry shouldn't use its consumerist immaturity, and lack of transparency and analytics as an excuse to inhibit, restrict, or delay outstanding customer service and outcomes. The market isn't going to tolerate it, and the winners will figure out a way to deliver it.

My concluding message here is that there is nothing less humanistic, professional, or ethical about helping a customer than treating a patient. I would argue that if we attend to our healthcare customers and truly serve them, then the sense of ourselves upholding professional, medical, and ethical principles is likely to take precedence. If anything, I believe that the conceptual frame of "patient" has held back our potential to deliver upon the mission of medical professionalism.

All aspects of care—including prevention, wellness, secondary prevention, and management of chronic disease—should be based on the foundation of our social, emotional, and existential lives as human beings. Our health—and therefore our healthcare—is not separate from these other parts of who we are. If anything, our health is a manifestation and a consequence of these and other factors. The Marketing Mindset provides us with a much richer conceptual frame, and the specific steps in which to understand the anatomy, physiology, and psychology of the healthcare customer/consumer, and not just the anatomy of their organs, the physiology of their clinical conditions and the psychology of their diseases.

In the next three sections of this book, we're going to dive into the steps of the consumer-centric Marketing Mindset with more specifics and examples.

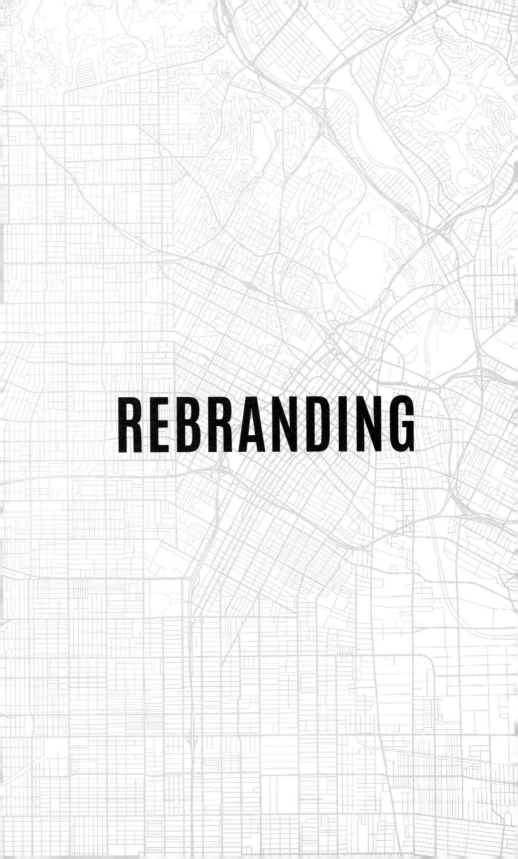

REBRANDING

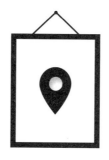

CHAPTER 4

REBRANDING

I've learned that people will forget what you said, people will forget what you did, but people will never forget how you made them feel.

—Maya Angelou, American poet, writer, and civil rights activist

Nothing about the Marketing Mindset approach—the rebranding, redesigning, and reorganizing—was critically needed by healthcare organizations, that is, until recently. Healthcare wasn't the hyper-competitive marketplace emerging today; and it most certainly wasn't customer-oriented. But times have already changed, and the shifting changes are accelerating. How well those of us in healthcare understand and execute the steps of the Marketing Mindset will make a significant difference for providers, organizations, and most importantly, healthcare customers.

I'd like to share an encouraging but realistic call-to-action by Peter Drucker, who wrote, "The greatest danger in times of turbulence is not the turbulence—it is to act with yesterday's logic." Building on this quote, let's remind ourselves of some current realities of the "turbulent" healthcare market—which we'll dive into much more deeply in the section on reorganizing. The healthcare market is anything but static, stable, or contained. It is in a chaotic state of tumultuous eruption and tectonic disruption. New entrants—from large corporations to smaller start-ups have the advantage of already deploying the Marketing Mindset in other industries. That is to say that the Marketing Mindset is not new to them. They now have to learn how to apply it to healthcare. These new entrants also have an advantage in not having to deconstruct legacy mindsets, such as the "patient" model that we discussed at great length in the previous chapter. For some, the "acting with today's logic" guideline presented in this book is going to seem natural. For others, it may seem as if I'm asking you to embrace something bizarre, fringe, or even irrelevant. If you choose to go down the reframe healthcare path, in whatever way you choose to adopt and adapt the Marketing Mindset reframe, at the very least you'll have shifted from yesterday's thinking into the mindset required to thrive in the future of healthcare.

Engaging the Marketing Mindset

The steps of the combined Reframe Roadmap and the Marketing Mindset are sequential and iterative. Once you reorient your thinking and redefine the problems to be solved, the next step—the first of the Marketing Mindset—is rebranding. Maya Angelou's profound statement about how you make people feel speaks to the essence of what a brand is all about.

A powerful brand is, at its core, about making people feel good about themselves in a specific context. Contrary to how most people perceive it, a brand is much more than a cool name, logo, symbol, color scheme, or jingle. It's an expression of the essence of the company and its products. As Simon Sinek popularized in his now-famous Ted Talk, customers don't just buy a product for its features (the "what"). Customers buy "why" it's being sold. Customers are even far less interested in the "how" of products.

> *A powerful brand is, at its core, about making people feel good about themselves in a specific context.*

People latch onto the why, which requires organizations to be explicit, clear, and consistent about the value of the product, the needs it serves, and the outcome or state that it delivers. This also means being clear about your target audience and your customer focus.

When I think about the basics of branding, the following two questions immediately come to mind.

1. Does your brand move people to feel remarkably differently and better about themselves and their lives?

2. In what specific ways does your brand make people feel better about themselves and their lives?

If you've read these questions and thought that the answer to question 1 is "No," you're in a great place to begin the branding or rebranding process. If your answer to question 1 is "Yes," then you're ready for question 2. If you are certain of the answer to question 2, you may be ready for the next step, the "Redesign" stage of the roadmap. There are other questions, but these are fundamental to me, and we'll cover some of the others along the way.

Earlier, I quoted Jeff Bezos. "Invention is not disruptive, only customer adoption is disruption." Why does this warrant being repeated? Branding is often misunderstood to be a creative or inventive activity. While branding does require some creativity, it's a limited understanding. Branding is a strategic, innovative and disruptive "must-do/can't-fail" effort. It is one of the most disruptive activities an organization can undertake, because it's all about setting a trajectory for customer adoption and retention of your services or products. People often confuse innovation with creativity or invention; but they're not the same. Creativity and invention are about making something new that people admire. Innovation is about making something new that people want and need. Your brand is your differentiating and disruptive attractor, your relevance and loyalty factor, and your growth engine. To consider branding as anything less than your core strategy is to place your endeavor at a competitive disadvantage. It's also a foundation for the next two steps—the redesign and reorganization of healthcare.

Branding experts assist boards, founders, CEOs, and senior-leadership teams figure out what their fundamental value proposition is and what core customer need is being addressed. That's not easy, but once a brand has been established, that brand is sacred. The brand goes way beyond any individual in the company, including the founder or CEO. If you have a solid brand, the whole becomes greater than the sum of its parts. The brand is a transcendent phenomenon, an iconic idea and message. Leaders who understand this also understand that the ongoing task is manifesting your brand—developing it, living it, promoting it, maintaining it and sustaining it. Like a garden, a brand

> *To consider branding as anything less than your core strategy is to place your endeavor at a competitive disadvantage.*

requires constant tending. At times, the weeds you remove from the garden are just as important as what you replant.

Determining a Brand

There is nothing "soft" about branding. This step of the Reframe Roadmap is probably the most challenging because branding is a deep-dive operation—and by deep, I mean emotionally deep. It is a deep dive into the human condition and psyche. The techniques to achieve branding are not as concrete as they are in redesigning and reorganizing. Rebranding is very much like storytelling about the heart and soul of the company and its customers. It's the step that companies tend to spend the least time on, but it is foundational. All the other steps emanate from the brand that you build.

At its core, branding is about meaning-making—perhaps one of the most unique and essential aspects of being human. Branding requires going beyond the internal workings of your corporation to clearly identify the external need(s) you are filling for your customers on multiple levels—the functional, emotional, relational, and existential. You can begin now to understand why the demand-side orientation is so critical, and why we spent so much time on it in the last chapter. These deeper levels of need touch core issues—trusting, social bonding, community building, surviving, and thriving.

THINK ABOUT SOME OF THE THINGS THAT HELP US TO SURVIVE AND THRIVE:

- Anything that makes us or saves us money or time or energy—physical and emotional energy.
- Anything that brings us closer to friends and family.
- Anything that contributes to a perceived sense of prestige and self-image.
- Anything that relieves us of stress, anxiety, pain and infirmity, and allows us to focus on other interests, activities, and people.
- Anything that brings us joy, laughter, happiness, and emotional fulfillment.
- Anything that makes us more effective or efficient in our activities of daily living, our work as well as recreational endeavors

In order to create a powerful brand, you must convey a clear sense of how your brand alleviates or prevents certain problems and pains; or offers opportunities for surviving and thriving.

AN INITIAL BRAND ASSESSMENT, WHICH COULD ALSO BE POSED AS A SERIES OF QUESTIONS, WOULD INCLUDE:

- what problem(s) you are solving for your customer

- what need(s) you are filling
- what tension(s) you are resolving
- what stressor(s) or frustration(s) you are relieving
- how you're making life easier, smoother, better
- how you're elevating their status and authority
- what capability or power you're giving them that they don't have now
- how you're going to make their time more productive and/or effective
- how you're going to enhance how others perceive them (at work and play)
- how you're going to help them feel better about themselves, their relationships, and their overall life

This list reinforces my previous point that the pursuit of consumer-centric healthcare is a humanistic endeavor. I encourage you to think of branding as an exercise in empathy. You are attempting to relate to people—to understand and to connect with the experiences and emotions of others. You are trying to assist them and support them in their life experiences. Branding, from my perspective, is not just a critical business step. It's one of the most relationally oriented activities a person or organization can pursue.

Think of a brand as sediment in the earth, and think of yourselves as "brand archeologists"—your job is to unearth the layers and levels of the brand. What archeologists typically uncover is below the surface level. Through their labor and skill, archeologists uncover more fascinating findings the deeper they dig. This branding archeologic exercise is difficult work, with very little glamour. But, the findings can alter our perception, understanding, and experience of ourselves in the world. Determining a brand should be like that.

Over the past few years, I have asked a question many times of myself and my colleagues during meetings: "If we are successful in this initiative or project we're working on, what is the specific outcome we're expecting, and how will we know (i.e. measure) that it's been achieved from the perspective of our customers?" There are typically two types of responses. One occasional response is that no one has thought it through, which means that we've been working away without a clear and explicit understanding of what we're trying to achieve for our customers. The second response, which is much more common, is that each individual on the work team has a different understanding of what we're trying to achieve. Without a clear, focused, and aligned understanding and articulation of your brand and its value proposition, it's difficult and confusing to engage in dialogue, let alone to plan efforts aimed at delivering value-laden services or products to your customers. It's like talking about a family vacation and trying to articulate what you're going to do and experience during that vacation without knowing your vacation destination.

As you work on your brand, remember that it's an iterative process. This means that you may spend time and effort working on rebranding, then move on to other stages like redesigning and reorganizing, only to discover that working on these later phases fills out or perhaps even alters your brand. That's not a problem or a flaw. The later phases, and your evolution, can very much inform the brand phase. That said, if you and your colleagues make branding an integral part of your everyday work, it will keep your activities and efforts well-focused. Let me illustrate an example of how rebranding might be informed and enhanced by a later phase. The following vignette is actually a combination of a number of advisory sessions with different companies that took a similar course.

BRAND ITERATION

I was advising a company that was in the middle of developing a new product. The session wasn't focused on branding at all—the group was well past that point. The purpose of the meeting was for me to respond to their product design, not their brand. As I observed the demos of their product prototype during the first hour of the presentation, I found myself becoming confused and bored.

One of their presenters stopped to ask, "So what do you think about what we've shared so far? Would you promote this?"

I responded, "Your product has some great features, and I think there are some real differentiators; but features don't sell a product. What I've been wondering about is what need does this fill for the people who would use it and for the companies that might purchase it for their employees?"

I looked around the room. Judging from the looks on people's faces, this was not the response they expected. They wanted me, understandably so, to tell them that their baby was beautiful. I couldn't do that. I had no idea what problem we were solving for. What fundamental contribution were we making? What core needs or desires were we addressing? I was clicking down the branding-assessment check-list in my head.

It was clear that they wanted me to respond to their product features: the cool screen layout, the advanced artificial-intelligence software and predictive analytics, the integrated suite of services. But

I knew that if there wasn't a clear brand promise, people wouldn't buy it—both figuratively and literally. They were swimming in the danger zone of the "consumer-also/supply-side perspective" and also, I thought to myself, in that danger zone of trying to be everything for everyone, everywhere, all the time. They hadn't brought me there to evaluate their brand, but I felt compelled to throw them what I considered to be a lifeline.

The questions flowed. "What need are you solving for? What is the outcome you're expecting to offer your customers?" I asked, with an intentional eye lock at each of the leaders in the room.

"We're giving them a tool to enhance their well-being," said the marketing lead, who was standing at the front of the room. "It's a wellness application with multiple channels and features."

As I looked at the confused and slightly frustrated expression on his face, I replied, "Yeah, I get that. But what if we weren't, for the moment, going to use those words 'wellness' or 'well-being.' How else might we describe the desired outcome?"

There were blank stares and fidgeting all around.

"Ok," I continued, "Here's what I'm hearing throughout your presentation. You've shared stories about how your other products are being used and the incredible outcomes they're creating for your customers. They're great stories, and they seem to be all about enhancing engagement. I'm not sure about 'wellness,' but it sounds to me like your product creates and facilitates engagement."

"Why is that distinction important?" asked one of the participants.

I responded, "We are talking about a product targeted at employers who want their employees to be engaged and productive. I'm not convinced that employers are all that interested in facilitating wellness, for wellness sake. It's an added bonus; but, if I'm an employer, I want my folks to be enthusiastic and need them to be engaged in their work. Right?"

Heads started to nod in agreement, and pens began to move across notepads as people jotted down their thoughts.

"Your stories imply that engaged and enthusiastic employees will be more productive. Loyalty goes up, turnover goes down; customer service goes up, sick leave goes down; health goes up and health-care costs go down. And look, employees themselves want to be engaged and enthusiastic. In fact, one could even define one aspect of 'wellness' at work as engagement and enthusiasm."

One of the product-development people piped up: "You're right. Our prototype customers were totally more engaged and more enthusiastic. But there was something else that really struck me about the change I noticed in them." She was now sitting forward and continued, "I think it was their energy." The minute the word "energy" came out of her mouth, you could see that she wanted to take it back. But a split second later, the room erupted. Three or four people began speaking at the same time. "Energy, yes, of course."

Like everyone else in the room, I found myself swept up in the engagement, enthusiasm—and energy—of that moment. One person called out, "The trifecta for employers—the triple E—engagement, enthusiasm, and energy." The room was buzzing, people talking over each other, others scribbling in their notepads and typing into their laptops. The lead person looked at the whiteboards hanging on the wall and said, "Let's remove that word—the one we've been using— 'wellness.' We're not calling it that right now. We are going to run with this idea of engagement, enthusiasm, and energy."

I sat back, took a deep breath and exhaled. It was exhilarating to see the difference in the folks around me, and to imagine the potential value we had just unearthed. The Reframe Roadmap and the Marketing Mindset had helped me to uncover their brand-value proposition. Now, to be honest, I had no vested interested in what specific brand they settled on. More important to me was that they now seemed to understand the questions that had to be asked and the issues to be addressed. Their brand would likely morph, and they might even return to incorporating the word "wellness." The one thing I was fairly confident of was that thinking about rebranding would now inform their design for the better. These small and rapid realizations could have a profound impact on every step to follow.

I turned to the person who had initially asked me what I thought about their product and whether I would feel good in promoting it to others. "A few minutes ago, I didn't think I could sell your 'wellness' or 'well-being' product, at least not the way it was framed. But I could definitely promote engagement, enthusiasm, and energy, and I believe your product meets those needs. I would pay a lot of money for engagement, enthusiasm, and energy; and I suspect so would a lot of employers."

Among other things, this story illuminates one critical point that branding experts talk about all the time. Customers are not buying products or features so much as they're purchasing feelings; or more aptly, they're choosing a brand that promises to create a specific feeling, emotion, relationship, situation or state of being. And feelings, emotions and relationships aren't commodities. Positive states of being are not commodities. They are, to quote a well-recognized brand phrase, "priceless." Core emotional and relational needs are priceless. If you can connect to one, you've got an incredibly powerful and sustainable brand.

Some readers may recall the iconic MasterCard ad campaign that was launched in 1997 and went on for nearly two decades—the "priceless" campaign.[33] It was one of the most brilliant, touching, and memorable marketing campaigns I have ever experienced. I distinctly remember that first television commercial, in which a father takes his eleven-year-old son to their first baseball game together. They walk through the mechanical turnstile for the first time; the father buys the tickets for himself and his son. He also buys hot dogs and an auto-graphed baseball for his son. The focus is on the transactions. During the commercial, there's warm background guitar-picking music and a folksy, relaxed voice-over announcing each item purchased and its cost: $28 for the tickets; $18 for the hotdogs, popcorn and soft drinks; $45 for the baseball. Final scene—we watch father and son sitting in the bleachers, shoulder to shoulder, just talking and laughing with one another. We, the audience, are bearing witness to a heartwarm-ing, archetypal, and coveted human experience—a father and son bonding. It's a timeless moment that tugs at our hearts. In the last few seconds of the commercial, the camera does a closeup on the son's face. He's looking up at his father—laughing and smiling. One can feel the affection between them, and you know, in that instant, that this will be one of the fondest memories that boy carries with him for the rest of his life. The voiceover's concluding remark, "Real conversation with eleven-year-old son … priceless. There are some things money can't buy. For everything else, there's MasterCard."

The entire commercial lasted thirty seconds, but the brand tagline emerged from months of detailed, in-depth, and qualita-tive customer research and field work. MasterCard listened to and studied its customers and discovered, to its surprise, that people were using their credit cards to purchase things for their families, to create experiences and moments like the one in that television commer-cial. It wasn't the transactional element or the business of making it easy to purchase something that was ultimately important to their customers. It was the ability to forge bonds, particularly with families and friends. It was about enhancing relationships and intimacy. The MasterCard campaign lasted two decades and became a meme in over two hundred countries across the globe! Their 2018 pivot to a new brand tagline was entitled, "Start something priceless." It sets lofty and far-ranging goals—targeting poverty, treating cancer, bringing more women into the tech industry, adopting pets, and educating our youth. The brand is still focused on a human need, but this time it addresses a different set of emotional, relational, and existential needs. This brand pivots around an expanded set of human needs: the need to give back, to help others, to be generous, and to be part of something bigger than oneself.

In both campaigns, MasterCard connects a surface-level, transactional need to a set of core human feelings, wishes, and values. Recall from chapter 3 the Kaiser Permanente brand tagline "Thrive" and the way it touches upon both a surface-level need and a core feeling. It's a powerful message, and it attracts and grips people, because it is so caring. Once again, I'd like to reinforce this understanding of the steps of the consumer-oriented Marketing Mindset as a deeply humanistic endeavor. I

Branding can be the ultimate exercise in expressing empathy.

don't know how to say it any other way: If done well, branding can be the ultimate exercise in expressing empathy.

Five Technical Principles to Help Clarify your Brand

Now that we've covered the foundation of branding, let's build on it with some technical principles that help achieve brand clarity. If potential customers have to spend time and energy attempting to understand or unravel your value proposition, then you have already lost them. People will not expend their precious time or mental energy trying to understand your brand.

1. COMPELLING STORYTELLING

One way that a brand can achieve clarity is by telling a focused story. Stories are constructed of specific elements that make them work. One example is the story where a relatable protagonist has a vision, mission, and goal; is confronted with a conflict, challenge, or antagonist to face down or overcome; and achieves a resolution or cathartic end. Stories have other elements such as unexpected twists and setbacks; experienced, wise mentors who guide, shepherd, and protect the protagonist; and archetypal lessons about life, the world, and existence. Storytelling-based branding is an art that health-care organizations must pay more attention to. Good brands, like good stories, are inspiring and compelling. I'd even go so far as to say that there is nothing as powerful as a great story if you want to create change in the world. Brand experts create stories that are not just speaking to your forebrain, your cognitive rational brain; they're speaking to and connecting with your amygdala, your limbic (emotional) system—the core of your primal being.

2. CONNECTION AND RELATIONSHIP BUILDING

A great brand builds connections and relationships. You have a relationship with a brand for lots of reasons—all of which are personal and meaningful to you. And when a brand resonates with you, you take it very seriously. This is the paradoxical thing about brands. Brands are less about a product or service, and more about the customer. The customer "finds" or "sees" him- or herself in the brand.

In this sense, brands are "see through." As in all relationships, the core is trust. If I decide to place my trust in the brand, and then the brand breaks that trust, the relationship is no longer pristine. It's hard to forgive and even harder to forget.

> This is the paradoxical thing about brands. Brands are less about a product or service, and more about the customer. The customer "finds" or "sees" him- or herself in the brand. In this sense, brands are "see through."

3. DIFFERENTIATION

One of the most interesting and unexpected things I've learned is that a brand does not have to represent something better. You must have value, and you must have quality, consistency, and reliability, but you don't necessarily have to be the best. For all the emphasis we place on producing things that are bigger, better, faster, and have more features, a brand is often more about being different that it is about being better. It's that differentiation that can attract people to your brand. We humans are neurologically wired to notice difference and change; it's embedded deep within our neurophysiology. PT Barnum—"the greatest showman"—said it much better, "No one ever made a difference by being like everyone else."

> A brand is often more about being different that it is about being better.

4. RELIABILITY

High quality is not enough; a sustainable brand also must be consistent. Your brand must have integrity. It must make a commitment on which it will deliver and that it will not break. The customer's relationship with the brand is sacred. Think about the brands that you continue to trust, love, and use. I'll bet dollars to donuts that they are consistent in whatever they deliver and however they deliver it. Brands that appeal to you have a reliability that is tangible. I think about how, when I'm travelling to foreign countries or even out of state, I always find myself looking for the brands that I trust. They provide me with comfort because they represent a familiar and reliable entity in an otherwise unfamiliar and unreliable environment. Good brands do that—they offer us a consistent, reliable, and protective haven in an otherwise inconsistent, unreliable, and unprotected world.

5. AUTHENTICITY

If your brand is lacking authenticity, it's going to end, probably sooner rather than later. The wisdom of the crowd can sniff out inauthenticity. Oftentimes a visionary leader and founder will create and contribute this sense of authenticity, but it must be sustained within every element of the organization. Iconic brands have compelling stories that are often written and told by the founder or CEO; but that authenticity must be recreated and reconfirmed by each successive leadership team, and it must be replicated and conveyed in every offering of the brand.

My hope is that this chapter has conveyed to you my primary point: great branding reflects and manifests the essence of our humanity. Great branding compels us to lead with empathy. It's not the icing on the cake. It's a core ingredient.

Great branding compels us to lead with empathy. It's not the icing on the cake. It's a core ingredient.

Rebranding Checklist

This checklist of items that create a great brand, along with the other guidelines outlined in this chapter, will assist you as you advance through the rebranding phase of the Reframe Roadmap.

- ✓ has a clear value: meets a need, solves a problem, offers a pleasure

- ✓ speaks to deep psychologic, primal needs and interests

- ✓ expresses empathy for those needs and interests

- ✓ is focused on how it makes people feel

- ✓ tells a story to which the customer relates with strong feeling

- ✓ establishes a relationship or makes a promise

- ✓ shows how it is different

- ✓ is conveyed with authenticity

CHAPTER 5

REBRANDING PRIMARY CARE

Misguidedly, many CEOs pursue the mass market when it would have been smarter to think smaller. This wrong-headed approach frequently happens in big companies, and the result is a watered-down value proposition that simply can't inspire brand love. If you want people to love what you stand for, you need to create products that are irresistible to a specific group... It's about products and services so targeted that they sparkle amid the clutter of an everything-to-everyone world.

—Jeremy Gutsche (The Proven Path to Unstoppable Ideas)

In the previous chapter, we discussed the why and the what of rebranding. In this chapter, we're going to move into the how. We're going to tackle a rebrand that's been necessary for a long time and that's already organically begun. What might primary care look like if we were to rebrand it?

It makes sense to begin the healthcare-rebranding process with primary care for a number of reasons. First, it's unlikely that we'll create great health outcomes and deliver accessible, affordable, and coordinated care without a solid primary-care foundation. Second, primary care is one of the most fundamentally flawed parts of our healthcare system, despite heroic efforts over the past couple of decades to change it. Third, by rebranding primary care, we'll address a significant portion of the larger healthcare problem, in part, because the model does include some subspecialty care. The larger point, though, is that if primary care is flawed, the rest of any healthcare delivery system is set up for failure.

Let's begin by picturing the typical primary-care practice. It may include physicians, nurse practitioners, physician assistants, nurses, medical assistants, referral coordinators, pharmacists, and support staff, all together in one practice. Each patient comes to this practice regardless of his or her specific problem, whether it's a hangnail, headache, or heart pain. Despite how different each individual patient's issues are, this one primary care practice is supposed to be everything for everyone, everywhere, all the time. But this construct struggles to provide highly effective, highly efficient, high-quality service in these wildly different domains of clinical care. It is not delivering the results it wants. It's not as cost-effective as it might be. It's not easily accessible, and it's not convenient. This is because it's a mash-up of multiple brands, and it just doesn't work effectively or efficiently!

That's not for lack of trying. We've tried to make it work for decades. Numerous iterations of this generic, primary care model have come and gone. Numerous generations of the so-called *primary-care medical home* or so-called *advanced medical home* have attempted to fix this model, without success. Rushika Fernandopulle, a Harvard trained primary-care internist, and CEO and founder of Iora Health, has a commentary which I believe applies here. He says, "you can't put wings on a car and call it an airplane." From a Marketing Mindset perspective, the overall brand and value propositions of the legacy generic primary-care model are too diffuse, unfocused, and diluted. There is tremendous brand confusion in primary care. While this may be taken as a criticism, another way to look at it is as an opportunity to unleash the tremendous potential locked up in primary care. The task at hand, in my opinion, is not to advance the current model; but instead to reorient our thinking and unearth its high-potential value through rebranding.

When we view things from a Marketing Mindset, we can observe that healthcare—specifically primary care—has already begun moving toward segmented brands. It's not a new concept, but it's not well understood, and therefore not appreciated as one of the most powerful underlying forces affecting how the healthcare market is rebranding and reorganizing itself. I have created a schematic of a potential rebrand architecture for primary care. This is less of a hypothesis and more of my observation—how I see the primary-care market evolving into a hyper-segmented, modular brand ecosystem—an interdependent delivery network of connected brands.

One of the underlying core elements of the Marketing Mindset is the concept of segmentation. This principle and approach is one that we already apply in healthcare; but we could apply it even more, and from a consumer, demand-side perspective. If we were to rebrand

I see the primary-care market evolving into a hyper-segmented, modular brand ecosystem—an interdependent delivery network of connected brands.

primary care using this principle of segmentation, we would discover five core brands, each of which carries sub-brands within it. We would also discover a sixth brand that I'm going to refer to as a "platform" brand. Like the others, the platform brand is composed of numerous sub-brands. But, unlike the others, the platform brand serves as a connector, a generative motherboard, an interface that integrates and coordinates all the other segmented brands.

I'm not overly concerned about whether there are five core brands or fifteen. This is an exercise in lumping and splitting—and a critically important one. I suspect and even hope that you will begin to draw out your own brand architecture. In the end, the customers and the market will settle upon an optimal formulation. The take-home point here is that healthcare needs to rebrand itself into segmented and hyper-segmented modular brands if we're going to transcend the significant limitations of the current system.

In the following pages, we'll consider each brand, its value proposition, its feasibility, and its viability.

On-Demand Urgent Care

The market has recognized a missing need in healthcare for on-demand urgent care (ODUC). Over the past few years, we've witnessed a rapid growth in the number of urgent care centers across the country. There has also been a smaller but steady increase in pharmacy retail chain clinics in CVS, Walgreens, Rite-Aid, and others; and there's likely more to come.[34] The ODUC sector offers a clear and focused brand promise, and for the most part, it doesn't attempt to dilute its business and clinical model with other primary-care brands. The value proposition narrative for the ODUC brand might go something like this. "Fix my problem fast. Make it easy to find, easy to get to,

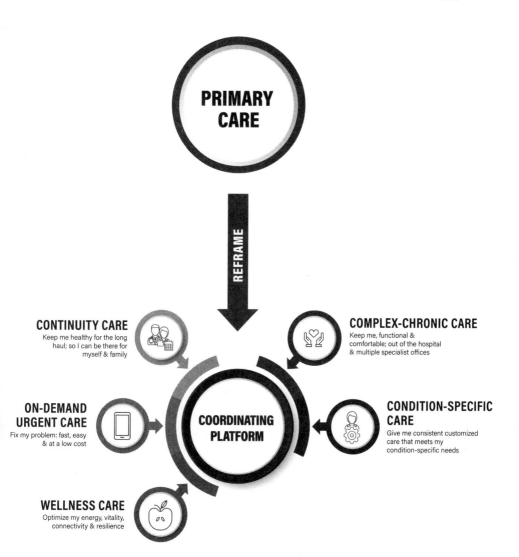

PRIMARY CARE ECOSYSTEM

Note: Pediatric Primary Care and Women's Health were not explicitly named but are a critical component of any primary care ecosystem.

easy to get in and out of. It should be convenient, low cost, with super customer service and fast turnaround time."

The first challenge or concern that arises regarding the ODUC brand is that primary-care providers believe this is a need they can fulfill. They feel that they already have an established relationship with the healthcare customer and therefore can offer greater value from an ODUC perspective. The dramatic market growth of this sector, however, reveals that customers perceive greater value in terms of convenience and time savings from a focused ODUC brand. From a cost-effectiveness perspective, ODUC doesn't require on-site physicians and therefore can deliver lower-cost care. Most models are now staffed by advanced-care practitioners with centralized physician oversight. There is greater operational and clinical efficiency within ODUC. Highly trained and focused advanced-care practitioners follow evidence-based protocols, so there is less unnecessary and costly variation in care. The efficiency, as well as effectiveness, is also a function of the limited menu of services offered and conditions treated in the ODUC brand. If all you do is attend to a handful of non-chronic, non-emergent conditions, you can become profoundly good at them. Contrast this with the generic primary-care office that can see literally hundreds of different conditions, from acute to chronic to highly complex.

The efficiency, as well as effectiveness, is also a function of the limited menu of services offered and conditions treated....

From a strategic and operational perspective, ODUC centers are more streamlined. Issues like wait times and turnaround times are paramount, so processes are limited, and technologies are also more focused and aligned, even down to the use of rapid online check-in, similar to what a client experiences at a hair salon or Starbucks. Because there is no need for chronic-care protocols or care-management technologies to be built into the electronic platform, ODUC can install lower-cost and easier-to-maintain databases, billing systems, and electronic medical records.

Customer satisfaction is also much simpler to operationalize and easier to improve, because the relationship is limited to a specific type of encounter. Numerous factors enter into play here. If you know that your entire scope of service is focused on urgent care, you hire providers and staff who are inclined toward, gifted in, and passionate about that sort of practice and healthcare-customer interaction. It's clearly not for every personality. The provider who wants a deep, long-term relationship with their healthcare clients, or is interested in managing complex medical issues, is not the right fit for this brand. Another factor that simplifies operations and enables better customer service is the issue of wait times. In a general primary-care practice, lower-acuity urgent visits can often be delayed by healthcare customers with more complicated conditions who require more time than scheduled, often unexpectedly. This highly variable exam-room time is something that the ODUC brand does not, for the most part, have to deal with. As an ODUC customer, you're not going to be sitting there waiting for an hour because a highly complex patient walked in before you and tied the provider up.

A focused ODUC brand facilitates aligned, effective, and efficient demand-side, customer-oriented service. One can also begin to appreciate how a focused, segmented brand allows you to better respond to the brand-assessment questions and more easily deploy the brand principles outlined in the previous chapter.

Complex-Chronic Care

The care of people with complex-chronic medical and psychoso-
cial problems involves a very small segment of the general population, about 2 percent. If you're looking at a population with a high
number of older people—those on Medicare, for example—it might
be as high as 5 percent. This small group of customers requires a
disproportionate amount of time and resources. The 2 percent could easily make up 30 to 40 percent of the total medical costs in a general population; and the 5 percent could easily consume over 50 percent of the costs in an older population

> ...the 5 percent could easily consume over 50 percent of the costs in an older population of patients.

of patients. This phenomenon—the disproportionate allocation of
resource utilization—was first described in the 1890s by an Italian
economist/mathematician named Vilfredo Pareto and has been
applied to numerous disciplines to explain distribution, consumption, resource utilization, and other naturally occurring phenomena.
The Pareto principle is often referred to as the "80/20 rule," which
in this case means that 80 percent of the costs can be attributed to
20 percent of any population. In the case of complex-chronic care,
extended time, money, staff, and other unique resources are all
necessary to provide appropriate clinical and customer-oriented care.
The care of people with complex-chronic medical and psychosocial
issues also requires greater connectivity across the continuum of care
and includes customers' families in a way that differs from other
primary-care brands.

Let's consider an example: Paul is an eighty-three-year-old man
with high blood pressure, obesity, Type 2 diabetes, and high choles-

terol who has congestive heart failure, and emphysema from years of smoking. He is, for the most part, wheelchair bound. He has had multiple surgical procedures including hip and knee replacements for severe degenerative joint disease and is partially blind due to a combination of glaucoma, cataracts, and diabetic retinal disease. Paul takes over a dozen different medications—many of which have side effects—and his ability to take these medications appropriately is unclear. He recently had a mini-stroke for which he was hospitalized. The hospital visit led to pneumonia and a blood clot in his leg, so he's now on blood thinners, which is dangerous given his poor balance and high risk of falling. He was initially discharged from the hospital to a nursing home, where he had to be treated for a urinary-tract infection, and after nearly three weeks there, he was transferred home with daily visits from a home-health nurse. As a result of his prolonged hospital and nursing-home stay, he lost muscle mass and is now weaker and more debilitated than when he went into the hospital. In the course of his hospital stay, he saw over half a dozen subspecialty consultants including a neurologist, endocrinologist, infectious disease doctor, pulmonologist, psychiatrist, rehab physician, and geriatrician. He was taken care of by well over a dozen different doctors and had many of his medications changed and doses adjusted. On top of his physical conditions, Paul is socially isolated and clinically depressed, which is greatly complicating his medical problems.

This is actually a very high level and superficial description, and probably doesn't convey the extent of the complexities here, but I'm hoping you get the picture. It's not just the breadth and depth of Paul's chronic diseases to which a clinical team must respond; there are also the complexities and consequences of severely limited activities of daily living, like walking, eating, going to the bathroom, and sleeping. And Paul's nutritional issues are of far more immediate relevance than in the other primary-care healthcare brands we've defined. If Paul ingests too much salt or sugar, he might end up back in the hospital in only three or four days' time. On the emotional and behavioral side, Paul's serious complex conditions and life situation, as was the case here, makes him much more vulnerable to social isolation, loneliness, and depression, as well as accelerated cognitive decline. Paul's care is further complicated by the need to constantly coordinate numerous specialists, identify issues around medical finances, and have difficult conversations regarding advanced directives, palliative care and hospice. Given the fragility and susceptibility of healthcare customers like Paul, clinicians and their staffs must be hypervigilant in ways that are not typical of the other brand segments of primary care.

Paul's case demonstrates several things. First, his needs are radically different from those of an urgent-care customer, or for that matter, a customer in any other primary-care brand. Given Paul's situation, we might say that the complex-chronic-care brand promise and value proposition must respond to something like this: "Keep me healthy enough so I don't end up in an emergency room, hospital, or ICU bed, or bouncing around between multiple specialists' offices. Keep me in my home and allow me to be as functional and capable as I can be. Keep me comfortable so I'm not in pain or undue distress. Enable me to live a life that maintains my dignity and that affords me the ability to participate in and enjoy interactions with family and friends."

Second, the chronic-complex-care customer requires a brand with a very different set of tactics, processes, and resources, with corresponding goals and metrics and a very different set of provider personalities. Not all primary-care providers are predisposed to deal with this sort of clinical and psychosocial complexity. Some have the knowledge, skill, and personality for this type of work; many do not. This sort of complexity also requires rigorously coordinated team-based care in a way that the other brands don't. For this brand, it really does take a village. The metrics here are radically different than in some of the other brands and include things like preventing inappropriate and avoidable hospitalizations; reducing

> *... the chronic-complex-care customer requires a brand with a very different set of tactics, processes, and resources ...*

emergency-department visits, specialty-care visits, and costly radiology testing; and eliminating medication-management errors. These are life-saving metrics and ones that, if they are carefully attended to, can reduce the vast majority of unwarranted and costly variation in healthcare.

Third, most primary-care physicians have a handful of customers of this complexity in their practices. An individual provider in a generic primary-care practice might become proficient at caring for this type of healthcare customer, but a practice devoted only to this type of care can become highly proficient and achieve far greater outcomes. It's the law of numbers and of scale: The greater number of anything a team does, the better they get at it. Practices and systems become more effective and efficient as the numbers increase. In a typical primary-care practice, it would be cost prohibitive to obtain and maintain the personnel and resources required for this type of complex care. But a focused brand can absolutely make the case for having specialized staff and resources. Even the exam rooms, office spaces, and electronic medical record need to be set up differently to accommodate this specific patient population and its needs.

Continuity Care

One way to think about this brand is to imagine the general primary-care practice with complex-chronic care and on-demand urgent care stripped away. This brand represents a primary-care practice that attends to customers for the long haul, from years to decades. The brand promise and value proposition are responsive to something like this: "I want a long-term, trusting relationship with a health professional. I want a medical expert who will be my health coach and health confidant for years to come. I want to feel assured that when I run into medical trouble, this experienced healthcare-insider—whom I know and trust, and who knows me—will be my personal clinical contractor and guide, helping me navigate the complexities of the system because he or she knows me well." It's a long-term commitment that this customer segment wants.

Relieved of ODUC encounters and complex-chronic care, this continuity-care brand can focus on primary and secondary preventive care. It can align its strategies, tactics, metrics, and resources to long-term, relationship-centered care. The providers who will be attracted to and selected for this brand are those whose personal style and passion are compatible with establishing long-term, trusting relationships with healthcare customers and their families. The brand will attract people who are interested in long-term chronic disease management, but not particularly in complex-chronic care. This brand does most closely represent our current-day primary-care practice. But, having said that, even within this brand, there are numerous potential sub-brand segmentations. For example, it might be that this brand includes a women's health sub-brand or a sub-brand devoted to people in their twenties or thirties who want an almost exclusively virtual and electronic relationship with their primary-care provider.

Condition-Specific Care

One way to understand this brand is as the entrance of sub-specialized care into the primary-care ecosystem. The brand promise can be articulated to meet this sort of need: "I have this one condition that I need someone to really specialize in and focus on; and I need customized, super-convenient, round-the-clock care and monitoring, as well as 24/7 on-demand response and intervention." By focusing on one condition, the entire brand can more fully understand and devote itself to customers' needs, their experiences, and their desired outcomes. The condition-specific-care brand, as the name suggests, is a sub-specialty primary-care model.

In reading the description of this brand value-proposition, one might reasonably ask, "Is all that really going to happen—24/7, specialized, customized, super-convenient, monitoring and responsiveness? Is this some futuristic notion?" The answer—which I'll go into later on this chapter—is that it already has happened, and so it's not futuristic. As with every other brand described in this chapter, this is not a hypothetical. It's already happening. These brands already exist. They are creating and unleashing new value by leveraging digital monitoring, automated responses, telehealth services, and machine-learning technologies.

Two factors have given birth to this brand. First, one driving factor for its emergence is the dramatic rise in the prevalence of chronic conditions. Conditions like diabetes, pre-metabolic syndrome, headaches, asthma, and depression are increasingly common. Thirty percent of the US population could be considered pre-metabolic, 10 percent have type 2 diabetes, and depression and anxiety disorders affect over 10 percent of the population. The prevalence and the rising costs of these chronic conditions have set up a demand for segmented brand solutions. The statistics on quality outcomes show that the current "primary-care medical home" model does a mediocre job of serving these specific conditions. It's no fault of the hard-working, bright, well-trained and mission-driven providers and staff. That generic brand of our legacy primary-care model is just too diffuse to allow for high-quality, customized care for so many different conditions. A second enabling factor behind the emergence of this brand category is the rapid and dramatic rise in digital health capabilities. These new, segmented, and condition-specific brand solutions can be delivered through a digital platform that leverages already existing, but rapidly advancing technologies such as machine learning, predictive analytics, automated responses, and chatbots.

Wellness Care

One largely unfilled need in our legacy healthcare system exists around wellness and well-being. The value proposition of this brand responds to something like this, "Assist me in staying safe, vital, energetic, and resilient. I want to be a high-performing, robust human being. I want to slow down the aging process and remain flexible and adaptive in body, mind, and spirit. Help me make the right choices and acquire healthful habits so I can be engaged, maintain high energy and the ability to learn, grow, adapt and contribute. I need to connect to my purpose in life, my sense of meaning and creativity, to master new situations in my environment, and to contribute to my family and community."

This brand is intentionally focused on keeping people healthy, well, and vital. Far from being merely a nice addition to the other brands, this brand is critical from a public-health and macro-economic perspective. Wellness and primary prevention are of global importance, but they appear to be reaching crisis-level significance in the US. There is a dire need for a wellness-care brand, supported by some dismal statistics.

> *There is a dire need for a wellness-care brand.*

A startling statistic from the National Center for Health Statistics (NCHS) of the Centers for Disease Control (CDC) is that, for the first time in recorded history, overall life expectancy in the US declined in both 2016 and 2017.[35] What's particularly disturbing is the degree of the decrease in longevity, and the fact that death rates increased significantly for those under sixty-five years old![36] Although some of this shift can be explained by the opioid epidemic, much of it is due to other social issues, including alcoholism, suicide, and the underlying socioeconomic challenges of poverty and joblessness. Some public-health officers and epidemiologists have even begun to refer to the increase in mortality in the US as "deaths of despair." In addition, these same researchers have noted that the disproportionate number of younger deaths have had a deleterious impact on the workforce and our economy.

The research and evidence supporting this brand domain deserves its own book. Fortunately, the wellness and positive-psychology movements have amassed tremendous knowledge and capabilities over the past few decades, as has the fitness, nutrition, and high-performance athlete movement. The sciences of habit formation and behavior change are also contributing to this brand category in unimaginable ways. Research on the social determinants of health, too, is of vital importance for this category. The fundamentals of food, housing, personal safety, safe neighborhoods, convenient transportation, accessible education, the opportunity to train for and be engaged in meaningful work, a strong community that enhances one's sense of self-respect, dignity, and purpose—all of these are integral related components of well-being and wellness care. The health of individuals, families, communities, and our public and economic health depend upon them.

One more thing to note about this particular brand. Recall the Pareto Principle, the 80/20 rule. In the case of wellness, the vast majority of the population requires this brand. Wellness is a relatively low-cost investment that yields great returns in both the short run and the long run.

Coordinating Platform

There is a concern among physicians and administrative leaders that segmentation of care will lead to fragmentation of care, especially insofar as these brands and sub-brands function as separate business units. This is where the "platform" brand comes in, as its purpose is to seamlessly connect the multiple brands and sub-brands by serving as a "motherboard" and stitching these interdependent brands together through data interfaces, analytics, and much more.

The coordinating-platform brand is made up of companies that serve multiple purposes including data interfaces, data management, analytics, predictive analytics, customer-relationship management, quality and medication safety management, health records, comprehensive electronic medical record keeping, billing and revenue-cycle management, care management, patient navigation, patient engagement, telehealth, other communication channels, and so on. As the primary-care ecosystem and the healthcare market becomes increasingly segmented, the need for interconnecting and interdependent support, or platform brands, will only accelerate. This transition will require coordinating platform brands that create value by serving to establish and maintain hyper-connectivity and hyper-collaboration across the interdependent network of hyper-segmented, value-adding brands.

Putting it All Together and Addressing Concerns

The five unique primary-care brands we've unearthed in this rebranded primary-care ecosystem have all been lumped together for decades, in a sort of undifferentiated "brand cluster." It's no wonder we're witnessing burnout in over 50 percent of primary-care providers. It's no wonder that fewer and fewer medical students and residents take up primary-care medicine. I believe the segmented brands that we've been outlining here have the potential to give greater focus to primary care and to provide a solid foundation for the transformation of healthcare delivery across the board.

I've heard primary-care physicians and administrators express three major concerns about this segmented primary care ecosystem. The first is the loss of the urgent-care visit within the primary-care workday. For many providers working in primary care, these encounters offer welcome relief from other more intensive and time-consuming visits. They also provide extra time for primary-care providers to catch up when they've fallen behind. The second concern is the loss of variety in daily practice. The third, closely related, is the loss of revenue to sub-brands and the loss of the role of the primary-care physician as the "quarterback" of the clinical team.

I believe these concerns are unwarranted. First, if we remove the truly complex-chronic care customers from the continuity-care brand, the daily schedule of that primary-care brand will be a lot more consistent and controllable, and the quick, less intense ODUC visits will not be necessary to maintain an on-time schedule. From an operations and efficiency perspective, there are tremendous gains to be had in this rebranded approach. Second, there is clearly plenty of variety and intellectual challenge in general medical practice, even in the absence of urgent-care and complex-chronic-care customers. Hundreds of conditions, thousands of medications, and the complexities of the healthcare system need to be understood and managed. Keeping up with the evidence-based literature alone here is a full-time job. I know firsthand how intellectually stimulating, challenging, and rewarding general primary care can be. Third, in the continuity-care brand that I've outlined, it truly is the case that primary-care physicians and other providers can assume the role of "quarterback" of the team—more so than in the current model. As the condition-specific care brand and wellness-care brand expand and evolve in the market, there will be an increased need for the continuity-care-brand provider and team to oversee, coordinate, and connect. There is a collaborative, symbiotic, and synergistic relationship between the condition-specific brands and the continuity-care brand. It is, as I've described, an interdependent network which will be connected through the platform-care brands. Healthcare customers are already availing themselves of these multiple brands, and I suspect that this will only continue. An individual customer might be participating in and simultaneously using a continuity-care brand as well as a condition-specific brand.

Finally—returning to the core demand-side orientation and customer-only principles of the Marketing Mindset—if this segmented interdependent approach is of greater value to the customer, we must lead with that.

Key Performance Indicators (KPIs) and Compensation

I have not made payment and compensation a primary focus of this book, but it is an important topic that must be aligned with any model of healthcare delivery. One advantage of the segmented rebranded primary-care ecosystem is that it simplifies and improves our ability to optimize and customize provider compensation. It's critically important to align payment and compensation with the type of provider behaviors and performance we'd like to see. In the current "mash-up" model of primary care, providers and clinical teams are measured on an almost impossibly diverse set of KPIs and metrics. Think about it: compensating providers for turnaround time would be essential in the ODUC brand, but clinically and ethically inappropriate, even deadly, in the complex-chronic-care brand. Compensating for deep empathy and long-term relational trust would be critically important in the continuity-care brand, but far less so in the ODUC brand. While some KPIs and metrics would cut across multiple brands, many would not.

Primary Care Rebranding is Already Happening

When I first began discussing this model years ago, people assumed that I was undertaking some sort of thought experiment. So, I modified the presentation by adding a PowerPoint slide. When I present now, I first show a slide with the simplified graphic or

schematic of the hyper-segmented primary-care ecosystem laid out—
the six brands. I then describe each brand as I've done in this chapter.
And then I ask the audience the question of whether or not they
believe this will happen. Increasingly, a larger percentage of hands go
up. But then I make a statement along the lines of, "We could discuss
the advantages and disadvantages of this rebranded primary care
ecosystem and spend a lot of time debating whether or not it will
happen. But the truth is that is already has!" I then click to the next
slide, with the names and logos of dozens of existing healthcare
companies overlaid on each one of the six brands. There typically is a
look of shock and awe on the faces of the audience members. I then
spend the rest of the presentation providing descriptions of a few of
the companies within each of the six brands. I'll mention below a few
of the currently existing organizations within each category, but a
more detailed description—that would do justice to the dozens, if
not hundreds, of healthcare companies within each brand—would
literally require another book.

So again, the reality is that the healthcare market has already
shifted and is rapidly redefining, rebranding, and reorganizing itself
into segmented and sub-segmented brands. In other words, the
question is not whether this will happen, but rather to what extent,
in what ways, and at what pace. There are dozens of segmented
and hyper-segmented companies within each brand category,
including within the platform brand. It's gotten to the point
where I can't keep up with the companies that are emerging in the

> *The reality is that the healthcare market has already shifted and is rapidly redefining, rebranding, and reorganizing itself into segmented and sub-segmented brands.*

advancing hyper-segmented primary-care ecosystem. I used to try to keep my PowerPoint slides up to date, but I've given up because the new market is advancing so rapidly.

Here are a few present-day examples. In the complex-chronic-care brand, there are companies such as Iora Health,[37] Care More, ChenMed,[38] Landmark and many others. Other sub-segments of this brand domain include nursing homes and the burgeoning home-healthcare space. There are a growing number of market-redefining provider groups that have emerged within the condition-specific-care brand, including Omada Health,[39] Virta,[40] SensorRx,[41] and Livongo—covering conditions like pre-diabetes, metabolic syndrome, diabetes type 2, migraine headaches, musculoskeletal issues, and behavioral health. Numerous Urgent Care and Retail Care venues already dominate in the ODUC brand domain; and I suspect that we are about to witness a second wave of disruptive innovation in the retail space.

The coordinating platform is an interesting and complex brand in that it crosses over all the other brands, and has profound reach and impact across the various segments of the population. Within this brand domain, there are game-changing companies such as Xealth,[42] Stanson, Patient Ping, Navihealth, as well as telehealth companies such as American Well, Teladoc, MDLive, and Doctor on Demand. There are literally hundreds of other companies within this brand domain, again, way too many to list here. The coordinating-platform brand is qualitatively different from the other brands because of its myriad of networking, connecting, analyzing, navigating, communicating, and facilitating value propositions that include and extend beyond the primary care ecosystem. This vast coordinating platform brand domain reminds me of the generative power of the Internet. As Steven Johnson put it in his book, *Where Good Ideas*

Come From, "There are good ideas, and then there are good ideas that make it easier to have other good ideas." The coordinating-platform brand fits into the latter generative category.

Summary

> *I consider the segmented rebranding and reorganizing of healthcare delivery to be one the most significant transformational shifts in healthcare delivery.*

I consider the segmented rebranding and reorganizing of healthcare delivery to be one the most significant transformational shifts in healthcare delivery. These focused brands perform with much greater effectiveness, efficiency, and sustainability. They can improve care outcomes, improve customer experience, and lower costs of care.

The Marketing Mindset reframe allows us to make sense of the rapidly emerging megatrends in healthcare. My hope is that you use the description of these patterns and the outline of the Marketing Mindset to discern and promote value-adding, demand-side trends from supply-side artifacts within your own organizations. My hope is that you use this knowledge to contribute to the advancement of value-based, customer-only care.

We've covered the rebranding of primary care in this chapter. In chapter 8, we'll go into greater detail on the reorganization of primary care—completing the full cycle of the Reframe Roadmap/Marketing Mindset. Again, it is imperative that we follow all the steps if we are to transform primary care and healthcare delivery overall.

Now, let's move onto the next step of the Marketing Mindset.

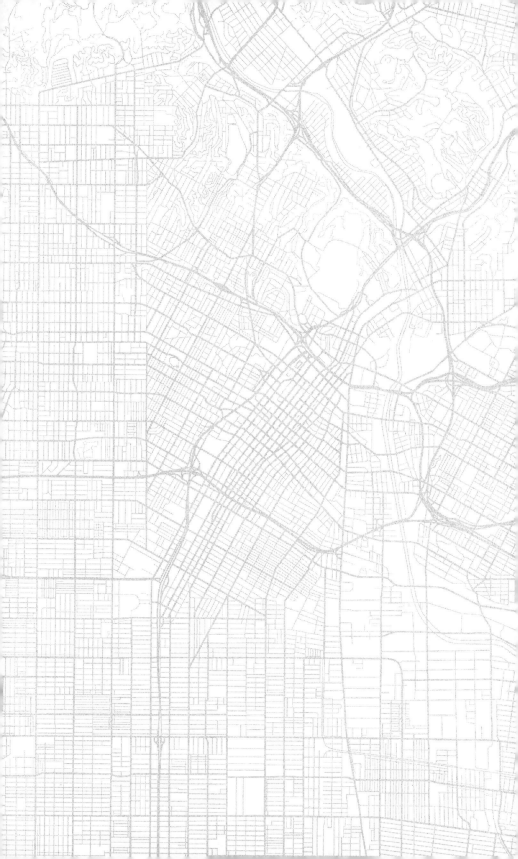

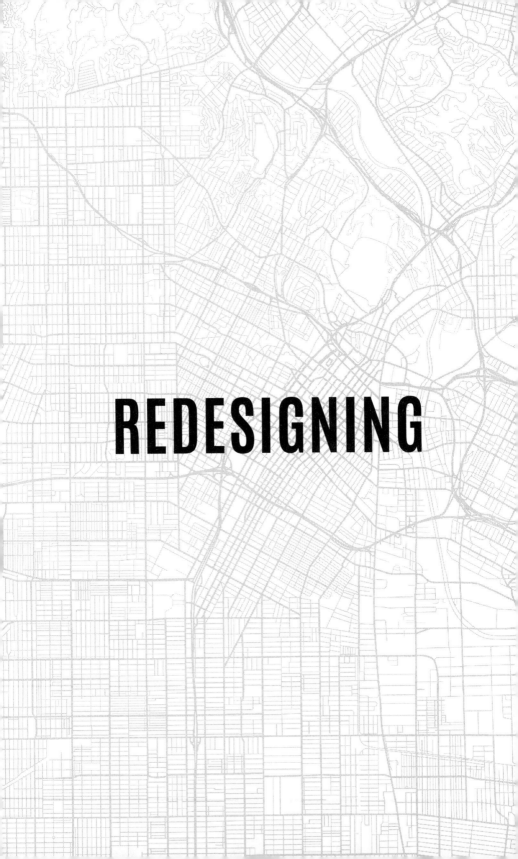

REDESIGNING

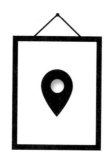

C H A P T E R   6

REDESIGNING

People talk about our healthcare system needing to be fixed.
The system isn't broken. It's just designed for the wrong thing.

— Marcus Osborne, VP of Health and Wellness, Walmart[43]

I believe that the consumer-oriented Marketing Mindset is the most advanced and comprehensive expression of empathy that we can introduce into healthcare today. It surpasses the current approaches to patient-centered care and advances the core ethos of the medical profession by systematically enabling a focused rebranding, redesigning, and reorganizing of healthcare around the needs of its customers.

> *Marketing Mindset is the most advanced and comprehensive expression of empathy that we can introduce into healthcare today.*

Our next step in applying the Marketing Mindset is to focus on design. Design thinking, with its myriad approaches, techniques, and technologies, is about nothing less than elevating the human experience and the human condition. From my perspective, a good design uplifts human existence in a way which is second only to human interaction and great storytelling.

Design thinking is about nothing less than elevating the human experience and human condition.

Good design leads to surprise, wonderment, enthusiasm, and delight. It can create a "wow" experience or an exalted state of being. When an object or structure is well designed, it can make us feel respected and even dignified. Conversely, when something is designed poorly— when it's complicated or clunky or difficult to use—we feel frustrated and even dis-respected, pained, or harmed. A good design gives us energy. A bad design saps our energy.

Design is an established discipline that is part of almost every facet of our lives as consumers. Many of us have little awareness of how much applied design thinking impacts our everyday activities, affects our behaviors, and changes how and what we experience. Think about each product you come into contact with each day, and your experience with them: the alarm, the toothbrush, the shower head, the shampoo bottle, your kitchen appliances; the car, train, or bus that takes you to work. Whether it's something you consume or something you use, all of it is intentionally—and hopefully expertly—designed.

It's not just tangible products that are intentionally designed, but our experiences are as well. When you go into a great theme park, for example, you might have the sense that your experience is designed, as little there is left to chance. The same is true when you go into a shopping mall or a grocery store; those experiences are carefully designed. The placement of everything (including those candy bars near the cashier) is focused around the experience designers intend you to have and the behaviors they want to elicit.

If we don't understand, appreciate, and incorporate design thinking into our delivery of healthcare, we will become design dinosaurs—that is, extinct. But, if we appropriately attend to and resource design thinking as part of our Marketing Mindset reframe, we'll have more than a fighting chance to maintain and even enhance our market relevance. Some have remarked that our current healthcare system has such a fundamentally flawed design that it will be incredibly difficult to fix from within. The necessary redesign is so huge, and it will take those of us in legacy healthcare too long to accomplish; thereby allowing new entrants, such as the retail giants, the opportunity and time to establish themselves as the dominant, well-designed customer-oriented healthcare option of choice.

I think the picture is a bit more complex than that. I believe we need to immediately and rapidly pursue the redesign process because it's the right thing to do for our healthcare customers—for improving their experience and outcomes. I also believe that we can get a leg up on and rapidly advance the redesign process if we pay careful attention to the principles of design. What follows in this section are some basics that are important for you to understand. I realize that most of us are not going to be working in design; but having this knowledge, in my opinion, provides leadership with a competitive advantage.

Design is a highly iterative process. You don't just decide to reframe, rebrand, redesign, and reorganize, and then pick up a pen and lay out a plan in an afternoon. It's a multi-year process. If we're going to leap into the redesign game, I think there are at least three major realities that are critically important for healthcare leaders and incumbent healthcare systems to understand about the Redesign phase of the Marketing Mindset approach.

1. **Redesign is a "must-do/can't-fail" competitive imperative.**

2. **Redesign must be approached from a customer-oriented, demand-side perspective.**

3. **Redesign tools, resources, and expertise abound, so we don't need to invent them.**

1. Redesign Is a Must-Do/Can't-Fail Competitive Imperative.

Design is as critically important to healthcare and the emerging healthcare market as digital or technological innovations. And it has a profound impact on the bottom line.

A groundbreaking, five-year study published by McKinsey & Company in 2018 investigated over 2 million pieces of financial data and one hundred thousand "deliberate design actions" deployed within three hundred companies.[44] The authors discovered four different design interventions that were most effective in increasing revenue and total returns. They grouped these four domains into the McKinsey Design Index (MDI), and then rated and ranked all three hundred companies against the metric of design commitment and execution. The four domains of the MDI are:

1. Tracking the impact of design just as rigorously as cost and revenue.

2. Putting customers first by talking with and listening to them throughout product and service development and deployment.

3. Embedding designers in cross-functional teams and incentivizing top design talent.

4. Encouraging research, early-stage prototyping, and iteration.

The conclusions of the McKinsey study demonstrate the financial power and importance of putting resources into design. Across the three separate industries they studied—medical technology, consumer goods, and retail banking—companies with a high, consistent, and comprehensive commitment to design and who were adept at operationalizing design principles experienced 32 percent greater revenue and 56 percent greater total returns to their shareholders. Companies that did well in all four domains had "soaring" revenues and returns as compared to those who scored in the bottom three quartiles. The difference in revenue and returns among the other three lower quartiles was negligible, underscoring the point that in order for design to really make a bottom-line impact, a company had to be "all-in."

QUESTIONS FOR SENIOR LEADERSHIP TEAMS:

- How would you rate yourself on the McKinsey Design Index?

- Are you meeting all four criteria? If not, how many are you meeting?

- Would you know how to begin deploying these four domains?

- Do you have any in-house expertise to assist you?
- Would you know where to find outside expertise?
- Are you really willing to "wait and see" what your competitors are doing in terms of design?

Contrary to what we in the healthcare profession may have believed in the past, design thinking is not superfluous; it's not something that merely makes things look or feel nicer. My claim in this chapter is that—following what has already occurred in other industries and given the increasingly competitive healthcare market—the deployment of design thinking and redesign is a "must-do/can't fail" imperative. All of the new entrants in healthcare, and many of the highly competitive legacy stakeholders, are already creating next-gen healthcare products and services solidly based in design thinking and its application. These companies embed design experts in their projects because they understand the impact good design has upon healthcare customers' behaviors and health outcomes, as well as on their companies' own bottom lines. In addition, design thinking can and should be applied to support one's internal stakeholders—the people delivering care—making it easier, more sustainable, and more efficient and effective.

There are three reasons for us to consider redesign a "must-do/can't fail" imperative in healthcare: (a) patients have become customers; (b) healthcare is shifting to a value-based payment model; and (c) design-focused competitors are already out there.

A. PATIENTS ARE TURNING INTO CUSTOMERS.

Payers have been talking about their "members" for decades but are now increasingly using the language and conceptual framework of customers and consumers. In fact, according to Steve Nelson, CEO of the United Health Group, payers are trying to catch up: "We're not stuck to the traditional ways, and so partnering with industries that might be further along in the consumer mindset, perhaps, can bring in new thinking..."[45] Another large national payer, Aetna, conducted a brilliant Inaugural Health Ambitions Study published in December 2017, and as a result of that study, Aetna's website now describes its core purpose as "Exploring how *consumers* achieve their health ambitions."[46] This is vastly different language and a radically different framing; Aetna is not talking about patients just being considered customers. Instead, it's completely turned itself around to acknowledge customers who are interested in health—that is healthcare customers. This is no subtle difference! Hospital systems, too, are trying to catch up with consumer-oriented design thinking. Executives from renowned hospital systems such as Dana Farber, Partners Health Care, Beth Israel Deaconess Medical Center in Boston, and Northwell in Long Island, are working on engaging consumers by focusing on creating new and better customer experiences for them.[47]

I'm sure you can think of, at least, a couple of stories, particularly in healthcare, where you experienced frustration or felt offended and angry—from a customer perspective. From my own experience, I can tell you that when it is frustrating or difficult, I feel disrespected. It's as if the provider or organization has said to me: "I don't want to create an experience for you that affords you the decency, dignity, and respect that you deserve as a human being." Experiences like that can turn us away from ever using a healthcare product or service again. But, if an experience makes you feel good about yourself, you are far more likely to return to that product or service, and to develop loyalty to it. As we discussed in the rebranding section, we stick with products and pay what's required because their value propositions go beyond the functional need and reach deep within our psyches. Consumers vote with their hearts, as well as with their feet.

To date, we have not predominantly designed healthcare from a customer point of view. We've designed it, as I mentioned in an earlier chapter, from an internal point of view, from our point of view as practitioners and healthcare professionals. We expect customers to use our products or services, and then blame and label them if they don't, with terms such as "compliance" and "adherence." Think about it: In what other industry do practitioners demonstrate thinking or use language that blames the customer for not utilizing their product or service? Could you imagine an executive product manager at Coca-Cola or any other retailer saying, "You know what? Those customers are so noncompliant. I told them they should drink Coca-Cola and they're not drinking it!" Participating in healthcare is not the same as buying a soft drink, but in both cases, it's not the customer's responsibility to sell themselves on it. It is our responsibility as providers to engage our customers in their healthcare. It is our job to make engaging in healthcare appealing, even enticing and entertaining, so that healthcare customers want and choose to participate. It is our job to make it easier, more convenient and more dignified. It is our job to make it a habit to be healthy. That's where design comes in.

> *It is our responsibility as providers to engage our customers in their healthcare.*

B. HEALTHCARE IS SHIFTING TO
A VALUE-BASED MODEL.

The second shift that's relevant to our adoption of design thinking is the transition of healthcare from a volume-driven, fee-for-service model to a value-based model, and an outcomes-driven orientation. In other words, healthcare has not traditionally been measured or paid as a function of its outcomes. But we are shifting to a model of payment where outcomes, quality, utilization, and cost matter more and more. In that market, how our customers behave and what they choose to do is going to be reflected in healthcare outcomes, and will matter to the viability of healthcare organizations far more than it has in the past. Patients will also increasingly act like consumers and will be voting with their wallets and their feet.

C. DESIGN-FOCUSED COMPETITORS
ARE ALREADY OUT THERE.

It used to be that there wasn't much choice in healthcare. No matter where a patient went, the experience was customer-agnostic or cus-tomer-unfriendly. That's no longer the case. There are emerging competitors out there who deeply understand the principles of design. And they're not just little startup companies. Some of them are the largest integrated delivery networks in the country. They've realized that if they don't start designing products and services that entice and engage their customers, someone else will. And they're far ahead of the pack in terms of design thinking and consumer experience. They're looking at results, looking at outcomes, looking at customer behaviors, and adapting themselves in real-time.

Let me share an insight from Dr. Steve Klasko, the CEO and president of Philadelphia-based, Jefferson Health. Dr. Klasko has argued that healthcare needs to have the same ease and appeal as an online-dating site. Millennials, he says, will not tolerate a healthcare system untouched by the consumer revolution. According to the statistics he shares: 92 percent of millennials expect to have complete, two-way electronic communication with their providers; 83 percent expect to have access to all of their health information online, just as with banking. Seventy-eight percent expect to have total access to their family and their own inpatient and hospital charts, to be able to see them at will; 70 percent expect online scheduling and the ability to compare pricing; and 55 percent expect to be able to discuss health-related topics and compare providers via social media. Klasko shows the need to streamline services, because millennial and younger generations expect quick, easy, convenient, and effortless healthcare.[48]

But it's not just the younger demographic who have these expectations. Increasingly, we are a consumerist society that expects to interact with the world the same way we interact with Amazon, Google, or Facebook. And frankly, we know that the most rapidly rising segment of the population using these contemporary communication methods is not the twenty- or thirty-somethings. It's the forty-, fifty-, sixty-, seventy-, and even eighty-somethings. Grandma knows how to use the Internet, don't make any mistake about it. So, although Klasko's claims are centered on millennials, I think we can extrapolate what he's saying to a much broader demographic.

> *We are a consumerist society that expects to interact with the world the same way we interact with Amazon, Google, or Facebook.*

Another forward-thinking CEO is Jeffrey Romoff, of the University of Pittsburgh Medical Center (UPMC)—one of the largest integrated delivery networks in the country. In 2018, he announced a $2 billion project to transform UPMC into "the Amazon of healthcare."[49] To make that happen, they're partnering with the likes of Microsoft—on the design of new hospitals, new technologies, and new digital strategies. Romoff claims that once they get going, anyone who's interested in healthcare—provider or patient—is going to want to come to UPMC, because they're going to knock it out of the park. Romoff, Klasko, and other bold, divergent-thinking leaders understand that it is their job to be customer-oriented.

2. Redesign Must Be Approached from a Consumer-Oriented, Demand-Side Perspective.

If you want to be competitive and successful; if you want customer growth, engagement, and loyalty; and if you want to retain your customers throughout their entire healthcare journey, then design must be approached and applied from a consumer-only perspective.

In chapter 3, we entertained the objection that healthcare was not intended to be the same sort of experience as Disneyland. But I'd like to return to thinking about Disneyland as an example of the way that its design process might actually be something of a model for healthcare. The chief consumer officer at InterMountain Health, Kevan Mabbutt, previously worked as head of global consumer insights at Disney. In that role, Mr. Mabbutt was responsible for all Disney theme parks, stores, and the online experience. After having spent over a year in healthcare, he's well-positioned to notice some of the major differences between how healthcare understands consumerism and how Disney understands and deploys consumerism. Mabbutt tells a story about these differences by comparing the lack of understanding of consumerism in healthcare to the focus on the consumer during the construction of the first Disney theme park in mainland China.[50] If healthcare professionals were building a theme park, he suggests, they might construct it based on their own ideas and past experiences, and then invite people into it. They might send out experience surveys and organize a few focus groups, asking questions like "How did we do? How did you like us?" They might even use that information to improve upon the experience of the park.

The approach Mabbutt and his Disney colleagues took was very different. Mabbutt looked at the theme park design, not from a Disney perspective, but from a Chinese-consumer perspective. Instead of starting with the idea of a theme park and of the Disney aesthetic, he and his team first spent months observing the Chinese people in their everyday lives. They used multiple ethnographic and qualitative research techniques to understand how the Chinese thought about, embedded, and experienced entertainment, relaxation, and vacation into their lives. This meant paying attention not only to what people did but also how they understood their experiences on an emotional and social level. Mabbutt and his team worked to understand not how the Chinese people could fit into their theme park, but rather how a Disney theme park could fit with the habits and needs of the Chinese people. Disney did not begin by focusing their design planning on the needs of their internal stakeholders, such as the theme-park executives, managers, and staff. They were focused on one stakeholder, the customer, taking a "customer-only" approach. It wasn't customer-centric or customer-oriented. It was customer-only.

3. Redesign Tools, Resources, and Expertise Abound, so We Don't Need to Reinvent Them.

There is no need to start from scratch if you want to begin incorporating design principles and applications into healthcare delivery. Healthcare professionals can partner and collaborate with others. We can access numerous demand-side design tools that already exist. There are a myriad of approaches and techniques available for purchase, consultation, and for training. One example of this and one specific area of design I find particularly compelling and critically important for healthcare is "behavior design."

B.J. Fogg, an expert on digital design and habit formation, and Kevin Volpp, a leading healthcare behavioral-economics expert, are two of the innovators in the behavior-design domain. Fogg is a Stanford psychology professor who, over the course of twenty years, has been studying, teaching, and applying cutting-edge, habit-forming design techniques into computer programs and software. He runs a lab at Stanford and consults for major tech giants and online retailers. Most of the other "habit" experts I've come across have borrowed heavily from Fogg's original work. Before Fogg entered the field, behavior had typically been thought of as having two components or levers—motivation and capability—that could be leveraged to get people to try something and then form a sustained behavior. Then Fogg came along and introduced a third major lever: Environmental cues or

> *There is no need to start from scratch if you want to begin incorporating design principles and applications into healthcare delivery.*

triggers. If you want someone to eat more fruit, placing an apple on their kitchen counter each morning, or a bowl of fruit in the office staff lounge, could trigger that behavior. If you want to exercise more, having your gym clothes laid out for you near the front door of your house, or seeing your gym bag in the front seat of your car after work, can trigger that activity. Websites, apps, online search engines, and online retailers all use triggers as part of their design.

Volpp and his colleagues at the University of Pennsylvania Center for Health Incentives and Behavior Economics (CHIBE) and the same university's "Nudge Unit"—led by Dr. Mitesh Patel—have expanded on design experience for providers and patients. One over-arching principle is what Volpp calls "choice architecture." It means that the user experience is designed to make some behaviors or choices more easily doable than others, thereby nudging people toward that behavior. This approach, within the choice architecture of behavioral economics, has been labelled "libertarian paternalism." It's an elegant and simple design approach, which allows for free choice but makes it easier for individuals to make the more appropriate choice, given the purpose or goal at hand.

As an example—despite a tremendous amount of communication and education, the providers at the University of Pennsylvania had a generic medication usage of somewhere around 60 to 70 percent with the goal being 100 percent. "Generics" are medications that are equally effective and as safe as brand name medications but cost much less. While the use of generics does not directly impact providers, it has a profound impact on healthcare customers, as well as employers and payers. Currently, medication costs can make up 20 to 40 percent of the total healthcare costs for a self-insured employer that is paying for their employees' healthcare, and the prohibitive costs of medications are one of the major reasons individuals choose not to fill their prescriptions. The impact of using brand name versus generic medications is profound, not only on the cost of care but also on very real health outcomes for individual patients.

So, Volpp and his colleagues made a simple design change in the choice architecture within the University of Pennsylvania's electronic medical record. When a doctor ordered any medication for the patient, the generic equivalent would automatically pop up as the primary choice to dispense. The provider still had a choice and could intentionally order a brand-name alternative; but that would take time, attention, and energy, all of which are in short supply in a busy provider's work day. Within three months, the choice-architecture design led to a generic prescribing rate of well over 90 percent—a rewarding and clinically relevant example of simple design principles applied effectively to healthcare.[51, 52]

Design is not just an add-on for the purpose of attracting customers to a product or service; design is integral to the product or service itself.

Again, my intention here is not to transform us all into design experts, but rather, to create awareness and to emphasize that redesign is a critical and necessary step in reframing healthcare delivery from a clinical, experiential, and financial perspective. Design is not just an add-on for the purpose of attracting customers to a product or service; design is integral to the product or service itself. It's my belief that in the near future, our design capabilities will be a major determinant of healthcare-customer growth and retention, as well as a major determinant of our ability to achieve competitive performance outcomes. In this chapter, we've covered the "why" and "what" of design, so now, let's consider some core principles of the "how."

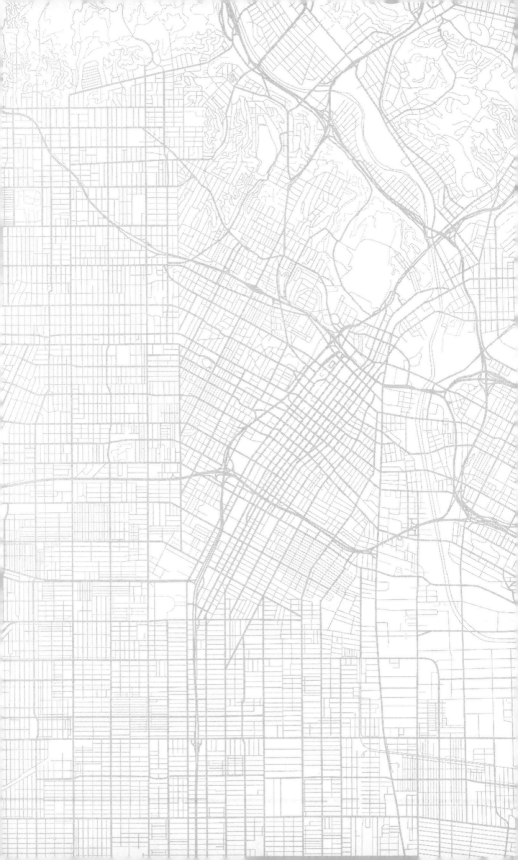

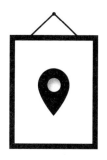

CHAPTER 7

PRINCIPLES OF REDESIGN

Design thinking is unlikely to become an exact science, but as with the quality movement, there is an opportunity to transform it from a black art into a systematically applied management approach.

—Tim Brown, CEO and president, IDEO

It wasn't that long ago that the quality and safety movement in healthcare was considered a fringe effort. It wasn't considered a core part of a provider's or hospital's responsibility to measure, monitor, and improve upon quality and safety. Fortunately, that mentality changed due to the courageous and brilliant efforts of visionary leaders in the healthcare quality and safety movement. Quality and safety are, without doubt, core competencies for any provider group, hospital system, or healthcare insurance company. Just as quality performance has become the price-of-admission, if you want to participate in healthcare delivery, I believe that design is rapidly emerging as a core competency. It's unlikely to become a regulatory issue, but it will determine success in the growing consumer-centric healthcare market.

My goal in this chapter is to assist you in cultivating a basic recognition and appreciation of these principles in order to evaluate the soundness of a design-based approach. I believe it will serve you well to understand these basic principles as you evaluate new products and services and make decisions that will profoundly impact your customers, your internal stakeholders, and your organizations. Here is a distillation of what I've gleaned from years of study, observation, and application. Please keep in mind that this is, by no means, a comprehensive list.

Nine Design Principles

1. **Design for Specific Target Segments**. Make segments as micro-niche as possible and focus them on the conditions and needs of the healthcare customer.

2. **Design for Outcomes but Love the Problem**. Design with the end result in mind. Move customers from reality A to reality B by resolving a deep issue that addresses a pain point, need, or creates an improved state of being.

3. **Design for Outcomes that Matter to Healthcare Customers**. Find out which outcomes and metrics matter most to your healthcare customers.

4. **Design by Starting with the Customer and Working Your Way Backward to the Product or Service**. This principle complements the previous two and focuses

primary attention and concern on healthcare customers instead of healthcare providers and teams.

5. **Design with Measurable Results and Outcomes in Mind**. Correlating metrics to outcomes that matter most to your healthcare customers will require that you consider new metrics for your new designs.

6. **Design for Simplicity and Ease of Use**. Complexity will sap your customers' energy, frustrate them, and turn them away. Aim not just to create ease of use but also to create delight.

7. **Design for Relevance and Engagement**. Recognize that different things are relevant to the customer, to the provider, to the clinical validation process, and to the clinical integration process. If you want people to become engaged and remain so, the design must be relevant to all of them.

8. **Design for Customization and Personalization**. Medical science is allowing us to personalize clinical treatment. The same is happening in the delivery of care.

9. **Design for the Behaviors You'd Like to Promote**. Use behavior-based design techniques that can influence the desired behavior.

#1: DESIGN FOR SPECIFIC TARGET SEGMENTS

Recall that one of the hallmarks of rebranding is segmentation. Although design principles are broadly generic, the actual outcomes, metrics, relevance, engagement, desired behaviors, and even the experience should be specific to the targeted segment. Design principles applied to the complex-chronic-care brand, for example, will lead to a very different design applied to the wellness-care brand. The principles applied within condition-specific diabetes care will yield a different design than those applied to asthma care. The more specific your target customer segment is, the more focused and customized your design decisions can be.

#2: DESIGN FOR OUTCOMES BUT LOVE THE PROBLEM

What I've observed is that most of us love solutions. We are seduced by the bright shiny objects, the promise of quick fixes, and the consultations that guarantee easy plug-and-play solutions. Successful entrepreneurs and innovators see the world differently. They are obsessed with determining and really exploring the primary problem. It's easy to get caught up in deploying initiatives, projects, programs, and technologies, but it's harder to clearly define the real problems and allow them to help us focus on outcomes. We'll truly be able to tell what we've achieved when we can distinguish and articulate an end goal and tell the difference between that and an intermediate goal.

We are seduced by the bright shiny objects, and the promise of quick fixes.

Roy Rosin, the chief innovation officer at the University of Pennsylvania School of Medicine states this principle simply and eloquently when he says, "You [must] fall in love with the problem. You don't [want to] fall in love with the solution."[53] If your sustained primary focus is on the end-goal outcomes, you have a better chance of falling in love with the problem and avoid being seduced by quick and easy fixes. One litmus test Roy shared with me is this: when focusing on the deeper problem, there are always unexpected discoveries or aha moments where you say, "I can't believe that! We never knew that before. Is that really true? How can that be?" Roy shared a story from working on the outcome of mobility, getting hospitalized patients out of bed early and often during their hospital stays to prevent negative comorbidities like muscle weakness and atrophy, balance problems, blood clots, bed sores, and so on. The team tasked with solving this problem discovered that many patients believed they were not allowed to get up out of bed or leave their rooms unless they were given explicit permission by the nursing or physician staff. The patients felt like they would be breaking hospital rules by getting up and walking around! This finding was completely unexpected and shocking to the research team—an aha moment—and gave them something new and different to build upon.

#3: DESIGN FOR OUTCOMES THAT MATTER TO HEALTHCARE CUSTOMERS

We need to design for outcomes that matter to our healthcare customers. What problems are *they* trying to solve? What are the pain points that bring them to you? Those are the outcomes that matter and that we have to identify very precisely.

Those of us on the provider side of healthcare delivery have our clinical and regulatory metrics of success, but healthcare customers likely have a completely different take on the outcomes that matter to them. In surgery, for example, we tend to measure things like the presence or absence of postsurgical infection or the number of days before patients can go home. These are clearly important and necessary outcomes, but they're not sufficient. The customer assumes that quality and safety are built in. The customer who has a total hip replacement expects the hip to work, and expects not to get an infection, a blood clot, or some other complication. What they want, however, is to be able to climb a flight of stairs, sleep through the night without waking up from pain, ride their bike, or dance with their spouse. Those are examples of outcomes that matter to the customer.

There's an International Coalition of Outcomes Health Measurements (ICOHM) that "brings together international teams of patients, physicians, and researchers to define outcomes that matter most to patients who live with different conditions."[54] To date, ICOHM has codified outcomes in nearly thirty "standard sets" ranging from diabetes to breast cancer, arthritis, heart disease, stroke, and for the "older person." For each condition, they've used tools validated in the medical literature to map out different domains that really matter to customers. These include issues such as: physical independence; the capacity for activities of daily living; energy and fatigue; body image; disfigurement; discomfort; sexual dysfunction; avoidance of medications with marked side effects like steroids; normal bowel habits; urinary incontinence; and so on. Their goal is to have these metrics adopted around the world. They have amassed an amazing body of work that is a wonderful example of this redesign principle in action.

#4: DESIGN BY STARTING WITH THE CUSTOMER AND WORKING YOUR WAY BACKWARD TO THE PRODUCT OR SERVICE

Every successful innovator and entrepreneur I have spoken to mentions this fundamental principle, which some have told me was popularized by Steve Jobs. Interestingly enough, it's also the first principle on the list of Amazon's fourteen "leadership principles." The specific Amazon leadership principle is called "Customer Obsession" and is described on Amazon's website: "Leaders start with the customer and work backwards. They work vigorously to earn and keep customer trust. Although leaders pay attention to competitors, they obsess over customers." Amazon goes on to say this about their leadership principles: "We use our Leadership Principles every day, whether we're discussing ideas for new projects or deciding on the best approach to solving a problem. It is just one of the things that makes Amazon peculiar."[55]

Aaron Martin, the chief digital-strategy officer at Providence St. Josephs in Seattle and a former executive vice president at Amazon, once told me why he thinks healthcare isn't currently designed for outcomes that matter to the customer. "The reason is, in the past, health care really hasn't been a B2C [business to customer] relationship. It's been a B2B [business to business] relationship. It's really been a relationship between government or private payers and the big healthcare systems. But that's changing now. Now the relationship has got to be between the consumer and the health system."[56]

I've heard a very similar perspective expressed by Kevan Mabbutt, Intermountain Health's chief consumer officer, who has had to defend the notion of the customer mindset to those who consider it less ethical or empathetic than the patient-centered mindset. Kevan has observed that the methods and approaches we use to improve patient-centered care can be unintentionally more industry-centric or provider-centric, than customer-centric. For example, our current patient experience/satisfaction surveys ask people to assist us in evaluating and improving our performance, as opposed to eliciting if we assisted our customers with their performance. He agrees that patient surveys have a role but argues that consumers' needs go beyond the clinical to the emotional, relational, practical, and financial, "and that comes from just listening to and understanding people." He goes on to add, "There's a lot of people who'll say, 'Okay, I get it, we've got it.

We've got patient advisory boards and committees.' But look... they have a role, but they're mostly just a sounding board to get feedback. They're not a prime source of insight that will really help us understand people's lives and how healthcare can be of greatest relevance." Kevan's expert message on this account is so important—"deeply understanding your consumer is where it has to start, and it has to be a continued focus... if we just did that one thing, everything else would work itself out."[57]

A similar viewpoint is also shared by Dr. Don Berwick, who is one of the groundbreaking leaders in the quality-improvement movement in healthcare. Berwick has said, "Listen to the patients. They have knowledge. This isn't about a focus group or the inclusion of one person on your board. It's not an interview. It's really getting the voice of the people you serve into the room, all the time, at every level. Always have the voice of the people you serve present."[58]

#5: DESIGN WITH MEASURABLE OUTCOMES AND RESULTS IN MIND

We have to design with results in mind and measure our outcomes. As the saying goes, "What doesn't get measured doesn't get done." To illustrate this point, let me tell you about Len D'Avolio, an assistant professor at the Harvard Medical School and the CEO of a start-up called Cyft.[59] He's an expert in biomedical informatics and analytics— what is now called "artificial intelligence." At Cyft, D'Avolio assists providers in predicting, with high accuracy, which healthcare customers might be at higher risk for bad events and poor health outcomes.

Healthcare often treats data as if it were exhaust instead of fuel.

Since his early days in healthcare, D'Avolio has been disturbed by the lack of data collection and measurement in healthcare and has used the metaphor that healthcare often treats data as if it were exhaust instead of fuel. His point is that we all too often let data be swept into the trash bin instead of collecting it and using it to improve healthcare delivery. He illustrates this point by sharing a story. Early on in his career, he was sitting across a lunch table from a urologist, a professor in the UCLA system. D'Avolio asked what he thought was a simple and easy question regarding one of the most common surgeries in the US—prostatectomies for men with benign prostatic hypertrophy. D'Avolio asked the surgeon how his results differed when he used different anatomic approaches for this one surgical procedure. The surgeon looked back at him with a blank stare. As it turned out, that surgeon—in fact, no surgeon—routinely collected outcomes data that were correlated to the approach taken. Keep in mind that this particular surgery is performed thousands of times each day across the country. D'Avolio had assumed that there would have been an automated, or at least, routine collection of data, so surgeons could study the data and understand which approach was superior. From his perspective as a data scientist, it was almost unfathomable that we wouldn't be collecting data that would allow for correlations to outcomes that mattered to patients, as well as surgeons. D'Avolio has a wonderful phrase that captures the situation for healthcare: "the field [healthcare] that counts the most, counts the least."

Len D'Avolio and his team create software programs that collect and utilize data, use algorithms to make predictions from that data, and then test out those predictions both retrospectively and pro-spectively. The programs can refine their own approach and their analytic capabilities as they "learn" from their own analysis of the data. It's the type of analytics that allows Netflix and Amazon to predict what movies you're likely to want to watch, and that allows search engines, digital-communications companies, retailers, and credit card companies to predict and act upon customized aspects of your life in their advertising and customer service. One final note when it comes to measuring for results: Len likes to remind me that these machine-learning tools are only useful as part of a concerted, multidisciplinary effort to affect change. Cyft, he emphatically states, is not a machine-learning company. It's a performance-improvement company that happens to use "artificial intelligence," because they represent the best tools available for uncovering what is actually working and pointing us in the direction of what we should be doing.

Another aspect of measurable results is the understanding that in developing new brands and designs, one must also be ready and willing to create new results. Oftentimes the legacy metrics used can limit and constrain new design. This is a challenging issue in that some of these constraining legacy metrics may be built into national performance benchmarks and regulatory requirements. There is much more that can be said about this, but the point is that rebranding and redesigning might also require reresulting.

#6: DESIGN FOR SIMPLICITY AND EASE OF USE

I had my first in-depth introduction to this topic in a book entitled, *The Laws of Simplicity* by John Maeda. Years later, Aaron Martin, the chief digital-strategy officer at Providence St. Josephs, helped me understand another one of Amazon's leadership principles called "innovate and simplify." This is third on the list of Amazon's fourteen principles.[60] What Aaron explained to me was that although it's relatively easy to innovate, it's far more difficult to both innovate and make something simpler.

Martin describes how Amazon simplified the publishing industry by splicing out all of the steps that made it costly and onerous for authors to get their books published and more difficult for readers to access those books. He describes his core design approach in healthcare as a transposition of this Amazon leadership principle. Providers of care create the value and healthcare customers consume it. He believes his job is to make it easier for providers to deliver care and easier for patients to obtain it.

A great example of the "innovate and simplify" principle in healthcare comes from my colleague, George McLendon, an accomplished scientist, professor, inventor, executive, and entrepreneur. Most recently, George has directed his talents to redesigning digital healthcare for migraine sufferers. There are and have been numerous digital headache diaries and apps on the market, but McLendon's is different, because, as he states, "people actually use it."[61] And the reason they use it is because he made it as painstakingly simple as he could. Let me explain. Over 50 percent of migraine sufferers underreport their symptoms to their doctors, and another 20 percent overreport them; so only about one-third are able to report symptoms accurately. One reason for underreporting is that migraine sufferers get so used to headaches that they typically only record the most severe ones, thereby underrepresenting the actual number of migraines they experience.

The problem with under-reporting is that the physicians then undertreat; and this leads to a vicious cycle of under-reporting, undertreatment, and prolonged suffering that can go on for years. The other reason that people underreport has to do with the design of the other apps and diaries that were available before McLendon created his. Most were too complicated and too time consuming to use regularly. In his initial months of customer discovery, McLendon learned that patients as well as physicians wanted a headache diary that was much simpler than the ones that existed. According to him, it's the simplicity of the app that gives it "stickiness" and enables there to be better and more accurate data for physicians to use when determining treatment.

McLendon made a surprising discovery which allowed him to simplify his design and distinguish it from others—one of his aha moments and a testament to the "love the problem, not the solution" principle. He learned that neurologists only needed the answers to four or five quick questions in order to decide on medications and dosing. As a result, his app is much easier and faster for the consumer to use. People experiencing a migraine can open the app and complete the questions in less than fifteen seconds and the physicians receive the appropriately limited amount of information they need in order to prescribe treatments that match the consumer's actual experience and need. McLendon's early results are revealing a marked improvement in accurate migraine reporting and treatment outcomes.

Elaborating on this principle of simplicity and design, Sean Duffy, CEO and co-founder of Omada, argues that the more painstaking effort you put into creating the best user experience, the less pain and effort the customer has to endure.[62] This principle applies broadly in healthcare. I've heard the same exact message from dozens of successful healthcare entrepreneurs. Designing for simplicity is designing for appeal. Customers should want to use your products and services and should come away not just with a feeling of health but with the sense of having had a healing experience. When design achieves simplicity, it

Good design feels like being known, appreciated, and respected.

hasn't just reduced friction and improved functionality. It has also fulfilled human needs on an emotional and existential level. Good design feels like being known, appreciated, and respected.

#7: DESIGN FOR RELEVANCE AND ENGAGEMENT

Specific questions need to be addressed in order to achieve design relevance in our products and services. A few examples include:

- Is the design relevant to the healthcare customer's life and needs?

- Does it touch the customer on multiple levels—functionally, emotionally, and socially?

- What specific problem does the design solve for the customer?

- Are our designs staying up to date with customer needs and expectations?

- How do we measure and monitor our continuing relevance and customer engagement?

- How do we maintain the connection to our customers as their needs and contexts change?

- Are our designs differentiating?

- Are our designs clinically relevant or validated?

- Is our design plan doable and sustainable within a larger context of other healthcare-delivery processes?

Sean Duffy points out that design "has to be relevant, otherwise you'll never have a chance. But even if it's clinically relevant, you have to provide the reason why people should shift their attention toward you, and that reason has to be interesting. You have to keep it new, fresh, and different. So, you're constantly thinking about how to communicate the value of your solution, how to continually make it engaging, and how to tell a story as people go through the whole experience. It's a marketing exercise, and you have to continuously sell the benefits and the value."[63]

It's no coincidence that Duffy uses the phrase, "marketing exercise" and raises the issue of story and narrative. Traditional marketing served only to showcase a product or service. Marketing for a bar of soap might show the soap and talk about how good it smelled, how fresh it made you feel, and how effectively it killed bacteria. Then along came a movement called "content marketing," so called because it led with new content that was not directly about the product or service being advertised. Instead of speaking directly and only about the product and its features, content marketing led with and offered a story that we could identify with, thereby engaging us as they wove the product or service into the story. I think of content marketing as storytelling marketing.

Storytelling has long been one of the most effective tools for influence, engagement, and behavior change. Recall the Kaiser Permanente (KP) brand proposition: "Thrive." To demonstrate their products and services, they literally show people thriving. One of their billboards shows a man jogging in front of power-producing windmills, and the line at the bottom of the billboard reads, "Increase Your Wind Power." It's a simple, powerful narrative, and one that invites identification on so many levels. Another billboard shows a photo of an older man with a basketball cradled under his

> *Storytelling has long been one of the most effective tools for influence, engagement, and behavior change.*

left arm; it reads, "Blood Pressure, You're Going Down." Again, a simple narrative that engages. They could have written something about the fact that KP can control blood pressure better than anyone else in the country, but they didn't go with feature-focused marketing. Another KP billboard demonstrating the power of narrative: an older man sits on a couch being bear-hugged by his two grandchildren. His smile is beaming; his eyes are closed. The caption reads, "Fewer Heart Attacks. More Hug Attacks." These KP billboards not only incorporate the principle of relevance and engagement, but also reflect the design principle of simplicity.

The thing about relevance and engagement is that it demonstrates how healthcare can become not only appealing but also enticing and entertaining. It demonstrates how good design can connect with us on an emotional, relational, and even existential level.

#8: DESIGN FOR CUSTOMIZATION AND PERSONALIZATION

In my opinion, the combination of customization, personalization, and individualization is the holy grail of design. There is no question that an individually tailored suit is a much better fit than one bought off the rack. The challenge—both in suits and in healthcare—is that personalization is costly, and most of us can't afford it. That's changing. In the digital era, customization and individualization are already happening. For example, as you scroll

The combination of customization, personalization, and individualization is the holy grail of design.

through online search engines, you've no doubt seen the type of ads that are customized for you. Digital advertising programs pick up what you're looking for and what you're interested in, and then push those products and topics to you. Online retailers like Amazon and Netflix inform you about what you're likely to need or like based on your previous selections. They actually get to know you better as you interact with them. And digital apps customize and personalize not only what, but also how they present content. There is no greater design than what is designed for you as an individual.

Medical science has followed a similar movement to what has been happening in retail. Dr. Eric Topol, for example, has been a brilliant and vocal proponent of what's come to be called "personalized medicine." The idea here is that we respond to treatment—whether for high blood pressure or cancer—based on our genetic makeup. We've known for years that certain medications work better in certain segments of the population due to genetics and physiology. But that specificity has now advanced to the level of the individual. Using genomic assays, we can tell if a medication will work in an individual, to what extent it will work, and even if it will be harmful. In some instances, like the use of anticoagulants, this has become almost standard practice. We know that some individuals have a genetic makeup for which specific anticoagulants don't work well. In the past, we had no way of knowing who those individuals were, but now, testing allows us to know if a specific anticoagulant medication will or won't work well in a specific person. Another example of personalized genomics is testing for the presence of the BRCA gene, which indicates that a woman is at increased risk for breast and ovarian cancer, and that a man is at increased risk for prostate cancer.

Continuing along the lines of personalized medicine is the concept of developing highly customized risk assessments for individuals. Some provider groups have begun to use electronic records coupled with other data and supercharged analytics to predict things like an individual customer's likelihood of getting Lyme disease or of having antibiotic resistance. Imagine just how personalized and preventive medical care could get if we could—with an individual's consent—combine health-record data, genomic data, and social-determinant data. It may sound a bit futuristic or overly intrusive, but large in-store and digital retailers, as well as credit card companies, have been utilizing a similar practice for years. They use multiple sources of personal information to predict what products customers need and want, with extraordinary precision. What if we turned that into healthful and preventive information? It could save lives in the hospital, as well as keep people out of the hospital by predicting those who are at high and rising risk for adverse events and outcomes.

The healthcare industry has also begun to introduce some design thinking at the population level, which is a great first step. Personalization and individualization will follow. Of course, customization and personalization are not entirely new in healthcare delivery. Individual physicians and surgeons have been practicing it for decades insofar as our professional training focuses on taking generic, evidence-based medical guidelines and applying those to individual patients. What's exciting and new is that these efforts are now supported both by technological advancements and by marketing techniques. Those that can excel at individualizing medicine and healthcare delivery will have a competitive advantage. More importantly, they will be that much better equipped to improve health and save lives.

#9: DESIGN FOR BEHAVIORS YOU'D LIKE TO PROMOTE

Dr. Dan Arieli is an internationally renowned psychologist who has written highly popular books such as *Predictably Irrational*. In a conversation we had about habit formation, I asked him what he considered to be the single most impactful lever for changing human behavior. His answer: how one's physical environment is designed and constructed. That makes good sense. If a stairway and a door are in a certain place, that's how you're going to get from one floor to another. Could you get there another way? Perhaps, but it's going to be a lot harder. The presence and absence of design, along with the quality of the design itself, makes certain behaviors much easier and more likely. If there are only fast-food venues in your neighborhood, that's what you're going to eat, especially if you're not able to cook for yourself. If your fridge is stocked with vegetables, fruits, and lean proteins, you're far more likely to eat a healthy diet, because that's how your behavior is designed.

Reframing behavior is one of the most exciting and impactful trends emerging in healthcare today. Our behavior, which has been shaped for decades by retailers like the food, automobile, and tech industries, is going to be increasingly designed and shaped for health purposes. The arrival of the digital-health platform is making this possibility much less costly and much more scalable. The digital-health revolution will serve as the enabler for what I believe will be one of the most significant trends in healthcare: behavioral design. We touched upon this at the end of the last chapter. The same behavior-design technology that's built into software games, apps, and websites can also be deployed within healthcare to improve customer adoption and sustainment of healthful products, services, and behaviors; enhance resilience; mitigate depression or anxiety; and change how we respond to stressful or unhealthful situations in our everyday life and work.

In the past, behavior change was believed to be a cognitive and rational endeavor. Our more current understanding is that behavior

> *Reframing behavior is one of the most exciting and impactful trends emerging in healthcare today.*

is far more multifaceted than that, involving neurophysiologic, emotional, and habitual determinants. As a result of this insight, researchers and clinicians are actively working on reframing the concept of behavior change. A brilliant example of bringing behavior change and design thinking together is revealed in the work of Dr. Kyra Bobinet, who has brought the methodology of design thinking together with applied behavioral and neuroscience. She explains that the field of neurophysiology is a pretty dry science that discovers and describes the neurochemical functioning of our brains and our bodies.[64] It predicts, on an anatomic and cellular level, why we feel and behave in certain ways and respond and react in other ways. The field of design, on the other hand, leans a bit more toward the creative and artistic; while the field of behavior change combines both qualitative and quantitative science. Bobinet has combined the neuropsychologic underpinnings of behavior with the science of behavior change and the art and science of design thinking. The combination is a powerful force, which she's learned to leverage and scale through digital health. By understanding how our brain works, Bobinet is able to design apps and other tools that elicit certain responses and that support people in creating and sustaining healthful behaviors.

A critical underlying principle of Bobinet's work is that she's redefined behavior from being something that one tries to motivate or force, to being something that we design, test, and iterate. This means that she approaches behavior as a continuous design process. What's elegant about her approach is that if the desired behavior doesn't occur, she says, "It's not you, the individual, who's failed; but instead a behavior design that just hasn't worked for you." The difference here isn't merely a mind game. It's actually a brain game that's critically important from a neurophysiologic perspective. Bobinet explains that there's an area of the brain called the habenula, which functions as a failure counter. When the habenula registers failure, it suppresses our motivation to do the same action again. From an evolutionary perspective, it's meant to keep us from repeating harmful activities. But when we want to change our behavior for the better, the habenula can be our worst enemy, lowering our motivation to try again.

Now, if the habenula doesn't perceive an attempt at healthful behavior as a failure, it won't inhibit you from trying again. Bobinet has applied this idea to an app called "Fresh Tri" that encourages users to build specific nutritional practices (or behavior designs) for themselves from a menu of crowdsourced habits that worked for others like them. The app continuously offers different approaches, so users can find a strategy that appeals to and works for them. And by framing each attempt as something other than a failure, this approach avoids the pitfalls of de-motivation instigated by the habenula. The app offers a non-judgmental and empowering way for the individual consumer to have control over his or her own behavior design and to normalize the notion that behavior change is not a single attempt but a continuous journey of redesign.

A Final Word on Design

The work of trained behavioralists, neuropsychologists, behavioral economists, software engineers, entrepreneurs, providers, and designers—now armed with increasingly sophisticated digital technologies, "artificial intelligence" software, and predictive analytics—has made behavior design a standard design principle. Without a working knowledge and purposeful deployment of behavioral tools, it's unlikely we will achieve the types of behavior change that are needed for healthcare consumers.

My hope is that the principles outlined in this chapter provide you with a foundational introductory base for understanding the power of design in developing consumer-centric, value-based programs and services; and in making healthcare more convenient, accessible, responsive, respectful, personalized, empathetic, and effective.

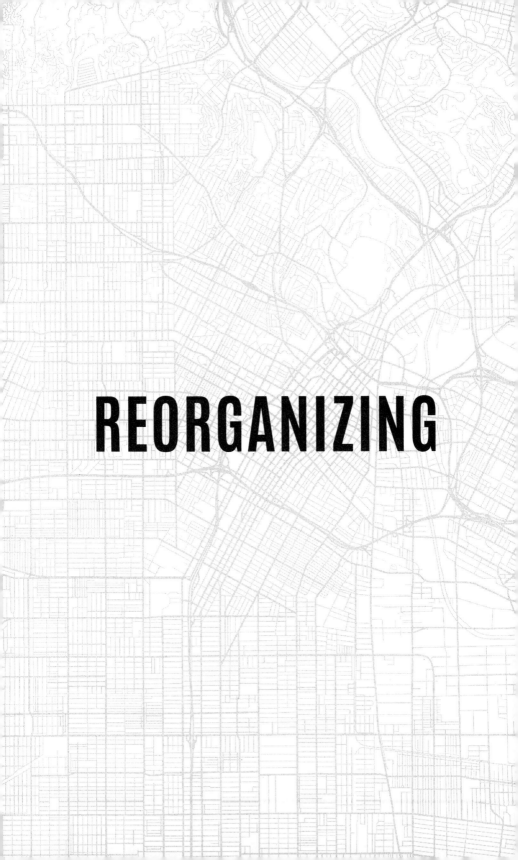

REORGANIZING

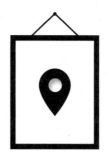

CHAPTER 8

REORGANIZING

...we're building a new model of care delivery... purely consumer centric, value-based, digital—all the things that it ought to be... We have worked with sponsors, because we have to get paid differently. So, we work with self-insured employers; we work with Medicare Advantage insurers; as we build this new primary care practice.

— **Rushika Fernandopulle, MD, CEO of Iora Health**

When I initially began formulating the Reframe Roadmap and Marketing Mindset, I was excited about all of the steps except, to be quite honest, reorganization. I understood this to be a critical part of the Marketing Mindset, but I thought, "Who can get worked up and passionate about reorganizing?" Well, I've had a major change of heart over the past couple of years. I now believe the reorganizing phase may be the most pivotal and innovative step of all. I never thought one could say "reorganization" and "innovation" in the same breath, but I have come to understand reorganization to be highly innovative—particularly in the current increasingly competitive and rapidly shifting healthcare marketplace. Reorganization may even rival digital advances in its disruptive potential, as well as in its potential to emancipate the value locked up in legacy structures.

> *I never thought one could say "reorganization" and "innovation" in the same breath.*

THERE ARE THREE CATEGORIES OF REORGANIZATION I WANT TO COVER IN THE NEXT TWO CHAPTERS:

1. Reorganization into segmented brands— The Primary-Care Ecosystem

2. Reorganization of healthcare systems into *health* systems

3. Reorganization through unconventional collaborations, partnerships, and joint ventures

Before we jump in, let's first review how we got to this final step of the Marketing Mindset. We began the Reframe Roadmap by *reorienting* our way of understanding the current state of healthcare. Then we set out *redefining* the challenges and the problems we are attempting to solve using this new orientation. Inserting the Marketing Mindset reframe, we engaged in *rebranding*, focusing on segmented customer populations and their needs. Armed with a specific value proposition, we then began *redesigning* from a demand-side, customer-oriented perspective—focusing on the results our customers want to achieve. The final steps include *reorganizing*, as well as *redirecting* our strategies, tactics, and resources.

Up until this point, all the steps have had to do with thinking in unconventional ways. *Reorienting* requires us to seek and adapt novel frames that are outside of our traditional domains. *Redefining* requires us to literally substitute the previous problems we're attempting to solve for new ones. *Rebranding* demands that we segment our approach and become highly empathetic story makers and storytellers. *Redesigning* forces us to think creatively and iteratively, with a focus on new *results* and metrics. Collectively, these steps also demand that we conduct enough research to understand and deliver on *results that matter to our customers*.

Compared to these previous steps, *reorganizing* appears somewhat concrete. It's a build and launch phase. These last steps— *reorganizing* and *redirecting*—are the means by which all of the intellectual effort and property that we've created up until now actually gets realized and manifested, and by which value propositions become value liberated.

> Reorganizing *and* redirecting *are the* means by which ... value propositions become value liberated.

If you do everything up until this step but don't manage to overcome your organizational inertia or gravity, you'll be left permanently stuck on the launch pad. It's the combination of these last steps—*reorganizing* and the *redirecting* of strategies, tactics, and resources—that allows you to avoid

> *If you do everything up until this step but don't manage to overcome your organizational inertia or gravity, you'll be left permanently stuck on the launch pad.*

being perpetually stuck in "pilot-phase" purgatory, unable to achieve large-scale, sustained change. Not following through on these steps can be demoralizing to the employees of an organization, because the promise of substantive change will be met with maintenance of the status quo. In order to progress forward, leadership must have the vision, courage, capability, and commitment to complete these final steps of the Reframe Roadmap and Marketing Mindset.

So, let's turn our attention to the first of the three reorganization categories. We'll spend the rest of this chapter on this first category and address the two remaining categories in chapter 9.

Reorganization into Segmented Brands— The Primary-Care Ecosystem

In chapter 5, we described how primary care is transitioning into a hyper-segmented, interdependent ecosystem. It's plain to see that this transition is going to require *reorganizing* the current construct of primary-care delivery. We outlined the reorganization of primary care into six major brands. We can think of these large brands as "brand families." For example, within the on-demand urgent care (ODUC) brand family, we have urgent-care centers, free-standing emergency departments, retail clinics, and other sub-brands. The ODUC brand family contains even more specialized or focused urgent-care centers like those for orthopedic urgent care, pediatric urgent care, and on-site employer clinics. In the *complex-chronic*-brand family, we observe numerous sub-brands— home healthcare offerings of many varieties, nursing-home care, rehabilitation facilities, transition services, and providers focused exclusively on complex-chronic and elder care. Because of the imperative for all these brands and sub-brands to be connected in order to deliver seamless care, the healthcare ecosystem will require an organizing and integrating platform. As we detailed in chapter 5, the value proposition of this *coordinating-platform* brand—also a family of brands—is that it serves to connect the other brands. Within the *coordinating-platform*-brand family, we see numerous sub-brands focused on a variety of different value propositions—from data collection and data interface, to analytics, to population health and care management, to predictive analytics, to customer-relationship management, and so on.

It wouldn't be optimal for these large brand families to function independently. Independent practices and networks of provider groups currently exist in the market. The problem is that they can lead to fragmented, uncoordinated, inefficient, and potentially unsafe care delivery. So, how would one envision the optimal connections, communications, and coordination between the brands? What I'm suggesting is a shift to something that looks more like an *interdependent delivery network*. What I'm suggesting—in contrast to independent delivery networks—is an open, *interdependent network* with seamless connectivity and coordination of care.

> What I'm suggesting is a shift to something that looks more like an interdependent delivery network.

Regina Herzlinger, the renowned Harvard Business School professor often referred to as the "Godmother" of consumer-driven healthcare, coined the term "focused healthcare factories" nearly twenty years ago.[65] As the name suggests, focused factories deliver highly specialized care for certain segments of patients. Her concept has some resemblance to the *condition-specific-care* brand that I've described. One might liken the primary-care ecosystem I've described to an interdependent federation of focused factory-like brands. I believe the reorganization we're observing in the primary-care ecosystem is, in some related way, an evolution of what Professor Herzlinger has outlined. It's also an evolution that relates to some of the seminal work on "integrated practice units" described by Professor Michael Porter and Professor Elizabeth Teisberg.[66] The emergence and potential market dominance of these focused and segmented brands is made more possible today, in part, by the advance of a digitally and analytically enabled *coordinating-platform*.

The transformation of healthcare delivery into a more broadly efficient, seamless, and customer-centric system will require a significant reorganization. An interdependent network model of segmented brands will not only be more effective and efficient; it will also be better aligned with a more transparent, open, agile and competitive marketplace—a market in which payment is based on transparent and measurable value.

THE NECESSITY OF REORGANIZING

There's an old saying: "No one likes a change except for a baby in a wet diaper," and that is no truer than when it comes to the process of reorganizing. In the Q&A sessions following my presentations on Reframing Healthcare, audience members often ask the following questions:

1. "Why can't we just rebrand and redesign, but keep our organizations and our practices the same?"

2. "Do we really need to reorganize to create optimal effectiveness, efficiency, and customer experience?"

3. "Can't we deliver on the promise of providing care for urgent-care on-demand needs, condition-specific needs,

wellness needs, and complex-chronic-care needs in our current organizational constructs?"

Here are my thoughts about these questions and the concerns expressed:

1. **The rapidly advancing market shift to segmented brands suggests that our traditional organizational constructs, particularly in primary-care, are not delivering optimal value.**

   We discussed this issue at some length in chapter 5, but let's consider these questions to illustrate the point.

   ▫ "How well can any legacy primary care practice know what its specific customer needs are?"

   ▫ "How does it measure if it's meeting those specific segmented needs?" (I'm not talking about general-patient-experience type issues, but rather, the specific customer-oriented outcomes and clinical needs that match each of the brand segments we outlined in chapter 5.)

   ▫ "How does the legacy primary-care model deliver the distinct value propositions of the various brand segments?"

   These are rhetorical questions, at least from my perspective. Despite decades of attempting to re-engineer, retrofit and advance the primary-care model, we continue to circle around a similar set of challenges, problems, and limitations. It's not just possible for one entity to provide outstanding care for all the brands we've defined; because each brand, as we articulated in chapter five, has a different brand promise, different strategy, different set of goals, different key-performance metrics, different processes and resource requirements, and different outcomes that it must deliver upon. No "one-stop-shop" primary-care practice model is going to be able to keep up with the hyper-competitive market of *condition-specific* brands, *complex-chronic-care* brands, or *on-demand urgent-care* brands, because these hyper-segmented and hyper-focused organizations will not only deliver markedly better performance and value, they will also be capable of innovating and advancing at a much more rapid pace. What is clear is that we need to reorganize.

2. **It does not make organizational sense to proceed with the existing model.**

    It is well accepted that the integrity, viability, and sustainability of any business model depends on the unique organizational structure that supports it. Any sustainable business model needs a specific vision and mission; a specific strategy that emerges from and leads to the fulfillment of that vision and mission; a specific set of goals and results; and a specific balanced scorecard to measure if all of the specific key performance indicators and desired outcomes are being met. Business models also require a specific set of resources— technologies, processes, and human resources, like people who have the affinity and skill set for that particular business. And any sustainable business requires a specific culture which, in part, guides how it motivates and incentivizes its employees. It's been said that culture eats strategy for lunch. Any business model has to create an ethos and a shared set of values that creates cohesion around and in-between all of the other parts of the organizational model.

You may have noticed that the word "specific" appeared in each cascading step of the business model—from vision to mission, to strategy and tactics, to goals, metrics, resources, culture, and incentives. If you try to mix the highly specific business and operational needs of a specific brand or business model, you'll violate its basic integrity, viability, and sustainability. What you'll get is a cacophonic mixture that will ultimately become ineffective, inefficient, and unsustainable. And that is precisely the problem we've been experiencing in primary care and healthcare in general. It's an organization problem in that we've intermingled different highly specific brands and business models. It's not an operational, human resource, technologic, payment, or compensation problem. I don't believe that value-based payment or pre-payment or digital technology or team building or stress reduction will solve this problem. And yet, those are the solutions we've been attempting to apply to primary care for decades. There is little one can do to fix the problem if you haven't rebranded, redesigned, and *reorganized* your healthcare business appropriately.

3. **This interdependent-network construct is much more enabling of agile, adaptive, and market-responsive brands.**

The current organizational construct is limited by the issue of suboptimization. In large, complex organizations there are certain processes and product lines that are prioritized. They are the ones most critical to the organization. As the

> *The current organizational construct is limited by the issue of suboptimization.*

organization works to optimize these processes and product lines, other product lines and processes must, of necessity, be suboptimized. That's the basic principle of suboptimization. It's neither good nor bad. It just is. There are always prioritized processes and products, because there are never enough resources to optimize everything. In healthcare, we see this rule playing out in large hospital-based, integrated-delivery networks. Generally speaking, what you see optimized in these organizations are the service lines with the highest profit margin—for example, orthopedics, neurosurgery, interventional cardiology and cardiac surgery; oncology; and perhaps one or two other surgical-based services. It would be a competitive disadvantage and financial misstep not to optimize these service lines. The investment in optimizing these services provides the highest returns, and there is also a very real customer demand and market/community need for these procedures and treatments.

As these few domains are being optimized, other areas, by necessity, become suboptimized. One specific domain that gets particularly suboptimized is—you guessed it—primary care. A major role that primary care plays in large, integrated-delivery networks throughout the country is to secure a patient/customer base and function as a channel for the high-volume, high-margin, hospital-based centers of excellence and ancillary services. Suboptimization is an unfortunate by-product of the way that healthcare is organized. In this organizational construct, primary care has, for years, had its value

> One specific domain that gets particularly sub-optimized is—you guessed it—primary care.

proposition sub-optimized, and its ability to perform and adapt in a customer-centric, hypercompetitive rapidly shifting market has been highly constrained.

The reorganization of primary care into a more autonomous, segmented, and interdependent ecosystem would enable these brands to optimize their value proposition and to be more agile, adaptive, and market responsive.

POPULATION HEALTH

Reorganization is not only consistent with a consumer-oriented free market; it's also consistent with what has been termed, "population health"—when an entity assumes responsibility and accountability for the outcomes of care (quality, safety, experience, and cost) for a specified population. This sort of situation exists for health-insurance companies whose products fully insure a "population" of healthcare customers, which is different from those that simply provide administrative services. These companies who take full risk or who have full-risk insurance products, assume a financial loss if the costs of care exceed the per-member payments they receive. They also have accountability for specific clinical outcomes of care and customer-experience metrics. A similar accountability and financial risk exists for self-insured employers that take responsibility through the provision of health benefits.

Some colleagues I've spoken with over the past couple of years seem to misunderstand population health as being less personalized care, but actually, the opposite is true. What population health means from an individual customer perspective is that providers, insurers, employers, and other payers are taking greater responsibility for outcomes—clinical outcomes, experience of care, and total costs of care. Deploying a population-health approach translates into an organization's assuming responsibility and accountability extending to every single individual in the population across the continuum of care and time. What this means is that the organization assumes accountability and responsibility for patients not just when they're being seen in the exam room, emergency department, or when they're hospitalized, but in their overall care.

In the pre-population-health era, an individual's first encounter with healthcare might easily be in the emergency department or some surgical or cardiac intervention suite. Within a population-health approach, it's the responsibility of the providers and payers to proactively identify and seek out individuals and make sure that their care is preventive and optimized. It's a win-win in that it makes good sense from a clinical perspective and from a financial perspective. It's a win-win in that it makes sense from the individual healthcare customer perspective and the system perspective. If the system that is accountable for population health withholds care or doesn't provide optimal care—especially for those who need it—it harms the individual and adversely impacts the system that is measured and paid on clinical outcomes and cost-effectiveness.

Some of the core capabilities required to provide good population health include the ability: (1) to identify all of the individuals an organization is responsible for; (2) to proactively identify and triage individuals by risk—low, moderate or high—for preventable conditions and worsening outcomes, and to also identify those whose risk is rising; (3) to assess whether the appropriate tests and treatments are being deployed; and (4) to track and measure outcomes, that is, to measure if people are getting healthier, getting appropriate care, and if the overall costs of care are optimized.

SEGMENTATION AS A STRATEGY FOR OPTIMIZATION

If you stop to think about it, the reorganization of primary-care into a segmented brands ecosystem is the optimal model for value-based population health. The various brands are hyper-focused on every segment of the population—from the *well* who want to stay that way, to those with *specific conditions* that require up-to-date, protocol-driven specialized care; to those at highest risk with *complex-chronic conditions*; and to the segment of the population that requires low-cost but fast and convenient *on-demand urgent care*. And the *platform-care* brand provides all the connecting and coordinating interface, analytics, and customer-facing technologies required.

> *The reorganization of primary-care into a segmented brands ecosystem is the optimal model for value-based population health.*

Increasingly, hospital systems and provider groups are taking on "population-health" responsibility—assuming contracted accountability and financial risk for the quality, cost, and experience outcomes of the populations they serve. These "populations" are typically groups of healthcare customers that come through government, private-payer insurance, and direct employer contracts. As the market shifts toward requiring this greater accountability—that is, as the market shifts to greater "population health"—we're seeing these organizations shift their focus to build or buy the specific brands and sub-brands we've outlined in the hyper-segmented primary-care ecosystem.

Some hospital-based and integrated-delivery systems are attempting to create segmentation within their current organizational constructs. As we discussed in chapter 5, the new entrants into healthcare have an advantage because they don't have to deconstruct a legacy of combined mash-up brands that have sub-optimized their value proposition. They're starting with a clean slate and can immediately organize themselves into hyper-segmented and hyper-focused care brands and sub-brands. The employers, insurance companies, and provider groups that realize the benefits of segmented brands and deploy this reorganization step soonest will be the ones in the most competitive position, allowing them to maintain the greatest scope of options. The organizations that postpone will inevitably be at a competitive disadvantage and continue to fall further behind.

There are several strategic options, or courses of action, regarding the hyper-segmented reorganization: *buy* all or some of the segmented primary-care brands; *build* all or some of these segmented primary-care brands; *outsource* and partner with segmented primary-care brands; *fully divest* of these segmented primary-care brands, and focus on other core capabilities; *partially divest* of some of these segmented primary-care brands; or maintain the status quo. Each one of these options has advantages and disadvantages. The only nonviable option, in my opinion, is to maintain the status quo. There are nuances in how one thinks about and develops these options, but a more in-depth discussion would require a greater understanding of the specific context of an organization and their market.

Summarizing this section—the healthcare marketplace is moving in the direction that will require reorganization, and with good reason. It's consistent with fundamental business principles; it's consistent with a consumerist, value-based open market. It's also consistent with the direction that other industries have been heading toward for decades. Most importantly, it's consistent with achieving the best healthcare system and optimal health outcomes.

FOLLOW THE MONEY—THE CAVEAT OF PAYMENT

Although the focus of this book is *not* on payment and payment reform, I believe it would be helpful to touch upon this issue in the context of the reorganizing step of the Marketing Mindset reframe. My friend and colleague, Tom Charland, CEO of Merchant Medicine and a nationally renowned expert in on-demand healthcare delivery, is fond of saying "You have to follow the money." He's right. Funding, payment, and compensation are the primary drivers of the way that healthcare delivery is organized and practiced in our country. Highly effective clinical models such as those I've described in the emerging segmented primary-care ecosystem must be accompanied by realistic payment structures, or else they cannot and will not be sustained.

It's clear that the current predominant system of payment—fee for service (FFS)—provides a perverse incentive to do more.

> *It's clear that the current predominant system of payment—fee for service (FFS)—provides a perverse incentive to do more.*

Payment largely flows from third-party payers (insurers) to providers. There are many ways to describe this model but labelling it an "open, free-market consumer-oriented system" is not one of them. This third-party, FFS payment model is one of the major contributors to the profound overutilization of healthcare that produces much harm (both clinically and financially) to individuals, families, employees, and municipalities, as well as to our nation's economy. It also creates obstacles to innovation and entrepreneurship, as any cost-saving innovation must go through the volume-promoting turnstile of this payment infrastructure. As we'll discover in chapter 9, this is one of the reasons that employers, some hybrid payer/provider (payvider) organizations, as well as some provider groups and individual practitioners are side-stepping the predominant FFS payment model entirely.

One way to resolve the payment dilemma is for the system at large to move to some sort of value/outcomes-based prepaid or capitated model, rather than paying for the volume of procedures, tests, visits, or hospitalizations delivered. It's important to note the advantages of a prepaid or capitated model that: (1) removes the incentive for providers to overutilize diagnostic tests, treatments, and referrals; (2) removes the need for unnecessary in-person visits, therefore freeing providers to interact with their patients in the most appropriate and consumer-centric way—whether that's by phone, secure text or email, tele-health virtual visits, or through digital apps—all of which create greater access of care and enhanced cost-effectiveness; (3) allows provider groups to optimally utilize and leverage their entire team of physicians, physicians assistants, nurses, medical assistants, health coaches, pharmacists, and others to create more convenient access, as well as improved cost-effectiveness and health outcomes; (4) incentivizes providers to focus on reducing preventable, high-cost care, such as ED visits and hospitalizations; and (5) allows providers to focus on care during key transitions, such as from hospital to nursing home to home healthcare.

There are clearly many advantages to prepaid or capitated primary care. Now, it does get a bit more complex in the specialties and with surgical care. And one major concern is that it incentivizes under-utilization, perhaps of sub-specialty care or of appropriate diagnostic testing. While this was a very real concern a couple of decades ago, it's much less so these days. That's because, as we discussed in the previous section on population health, there are countermeasures that have been put into place to assure that appropriate high-quality, safe care is being delivered. All value-based programs use population health and quality analytic platforms to track metrics such as ED visits, hospitalizations, care-gap closures, and appropriate chronic-disease-management processes, as well as patient experience.

This understanding—that an outcomes-based prepaid approach is far superior to FFS—does not fall in the realm of healthcare-related partisan politics. It's accepted on both sides of the aisle at all levels of government, and even more so in the commercial sector. We're seeing this realization demonstrated in the rapid adoption of Medicare Advantage contracts and Medicaid Managed Care (both prepaid-payment models). The prepaid approach is also the ultimate goal of the Medicare Shared Savings Program (MSSP), bundled payment programs, and the hundreds of Accountable Care Organizations (ACO's) and Clinical Integration Networks (CIN's) that have been created across the country. We're also seeing this demonstrated on the employer side with bundled-payment programs, direct prepaid primary care (DPC), and direct-to-employer contracts. To some degree, this prepaid movement has been accelerated by the rising percentage of self-insured employers who are now accountable for their own costs of care; and who are now incentivized to innovate their approach to healthcare benefits and employee health programs.

Now, just to be clear. Prepaid or capitated payment does not imply a single-payer system. What I'm referring to here is simply a shift to true, value-based payment—prepaid or fully capitated.

We're currently, in the US, in the midst of a slow and painful transition to prepaid/capitated healthcare. The MSSP, bundled-payment, ACO, and CIN models are all interim or partial-risk models. Their purpose is to ease our system to a full-risk, prepaid model. While directionally correct, these partial-risk programs add tremendous bureaucratic complications and costs while presenting some major challenges to providers and hospital systems. It's like having one foot on the dock and the other foot on the boat, with a strong wind blowing. Provider groups and hospital systems are trying to optimize and maintain their lucrative FFS payment revenue streams while also getting ready to shove off to more cost-effective, risk-based and/or prepaid payment models. It's a challenging and compromising position to be in, and it's unclear how long we'll be in this state of transition.

No matter what payment model we find ourselves in over the next few years, the Reframe Roadmap and Marketing Mindset remain critically important and relevant. In large part because our society and the market are bullishly consumerist and pulling healthcare rapidly in that direction. Waiting on payment reform makes little sense, and maintaining a status quo approach—that is, not adopting a segmented reorganization—will likely place any system at a competitive disadvantage.

Not adopting a segmented reorganization will likely place any system at a competitive disadvantage.

From a transformational perspective, a switch in payment from FFS to prepaid capitation will, in and of itself, not be enough to create a healthcare system that is consumerist, clinically effective, and cost-effective. The value-enhancing steps of rebranding, redesigning, and reorganizing will all be required to fully realize the benefits of any prepaid model. We have witnessed prepaid capitated models in other countries around the world that do not appear to be functioning well. It's my belief that these capitated systems have not been optimized, because they have not deployed the steps and principles of the Reframe Roadmap and Marketing Mindset and have not shifted to a segmented primary care ecosystem.

Just to come full circle here, the reorganizations that I've mentioned are not occurring outside of the influence of the realities of payment; but are, instead, occurring within and in response to the current payment system. They're happening because of the value-based disruption in the market, including payment disruption. So, I am following my friend Tom's advice. I am following the money. And the money is heading toward value-based, customer-oriented health-care—not just because it's more ethical, more affordable, and better care with better outcomes. The money is heading in this direction because it's better business.

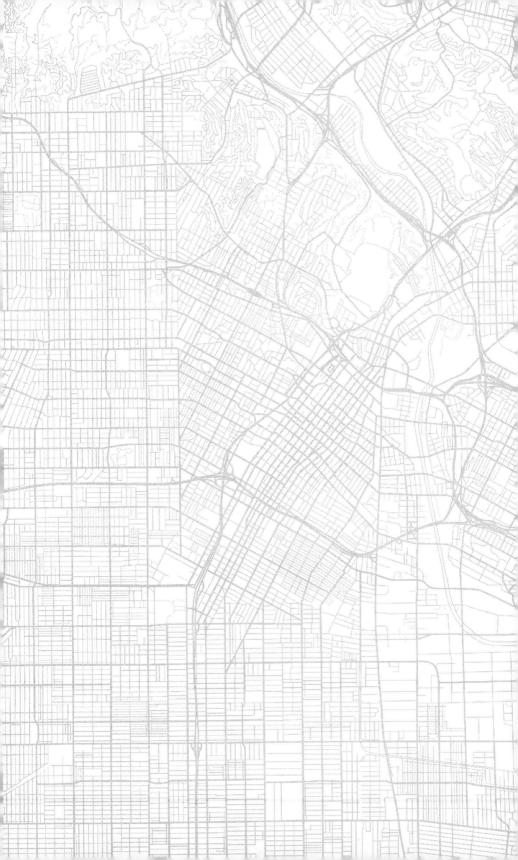

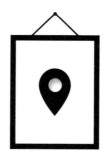

CHAPTER 9

THE DISRUPTIVE POTENTIAL OF REORGANIZING

*It's actually very difficult to change some of these structures.
My first emotional experience was, "wow there's so
many things that are messed up; we can fix these with
technology." Then I realized, "oh, there's actually a reason
why nothing has changed for the past few decades."*

—Sami Inkinen, CEO of Virta Health[67]

In addition to the reorganization toward a hyper-segmented, interdependent network of primary care brands, there are two other highly innovative categories of reorganization that are changing the landscape of healthcare delivery and greatly influencing market forces. One is the reorganization away from healthcare and toward a focus on health. The other is the growth of unique partnerships among previously separated stakeholders. The traditional legacy organizational lines are dissolving, and new, larger multi-asset corporate stakeholders are emerging. In this chapter, we'll explore these two types of innovative reorganizations, with illustrative examples that will provide us with a sense of what's happening and of what's to come.

Reorganization of Healthcare Systems into *Health* Systems

In addition to having the opportunity to interview Kevan Mabbutt, chief consumer officer at Intermountain Health and former chief of global consumer insights at Disney, I've also had the privilege of interviewing Mark Briesacher, Intermountain's chief clinical executive. The senior leadership team at Intermountain Health has, within the past couple of years under CEO Marc Harrison's visionary and consumer-oriented stewardship, initiated a bold move to reorganize itself into two entities: an "Episodic-Care" organization, and a "Community-Care" organization.[68]

The *episodic-care* brand encompasses hospital-based and procedure-based medical interventions. This includes all surgical procedures, whether ambulatory or hospital-based, including the treatment of trauma and acute events like strokes and heart attacks. This brand basically encompasses all acute and life-threatening pulmonary, cardiac, neurologic, endocrinologic, musculoskeletal, and infectious conditions. It includes medical care provided in hospitals, intensive-care units, operating rooms, and interventional suites. The *community-care* brand encompasses all the non-hospital, community-based preventive, chronic-disease management, and on-demand urgent-care brands—from primary care to specialty care along with their community-care services and partnerships.

This significant reorganization is a remarkably forward-thinking and courageous move. It takes real leadership at all levels of the organization. It takes fortitude and commitment. And, it takes a lot of hard work by a lot of dedicated professionals. It also takes a lot of trust among the clinicians and staff—within and across entire divisions. The amount of reorganization and self-inflicted disruption is profound. It's a great example of walking the talk. Intermountain's decision to rebrand and reorganize in this way is based on an intentional and thorough assessment of what their communities needed. Dr. Briesacher explained this a bit further, "So, we made the decision to move away from the traditional regional organization of our healthcare delivery system, and to actually reorganize around our patients, and around their families, the people that trust us and honor us with the privilege of supporting them and their health."

Freed up from their prior integration, each entity can now optimally deliver on its brand promise. The community-care brand can focus on proactive and preventive longitudinal care. It's unfettered and undiluted goal will be to keep people as healthy as possible, out of the hospital and acute-care settings. It will partner with other community stakeholders and resources to become an embedded and trusted steward of health in the community. In other words, it will have shifted away from healthcare, specifically acute healthcare, toward health. The episodic-care brand, on the other hand, can focus on achieving outstanding outcomes in its intensive, time-limited treatments and case-based surgical and specialty procedures. It will focus, unfettered and undiluted, on delivering effective and efficient high-tech/high-touch care and assure the appropriate utilization of these services.

One point I did not appreciate, until my conversation with Briesacher, is how synergistic and supportive these two large brands are of one another. As he helped me understand, "When you deliver on an episodic basis—safe, high quality care that's also affordable—that helps the people who are working on taking care of populations. And the work caring for populations, in terms of maintaining and advancing health or regaining health; well, that benefits our specialty-based colleagues when someone has to be hospitalized or has an acute condition."

There are obviously many other initiatives that Intermountain is engaged in—such as advancing its consumer orientation and digital-health strategies. But without this critical step of reorganizing, Intermountain Health would not be able to optimally carry forward its vision of delivering the highest-caliber community and episodic care. As Briesacher put it, "we can't hide behind the complexity of healthcare. You have to disrupt yourselves to get to the next place, and we're all in on that."

> "We can't hide behind the complexity of healthcare. You have to disrupt yourselves to get to the next place, and we're all in on that."

Reorganization through Unconventional Collaborations, Partnerships, and Joint Ventures

Over the past few years, a trend has emerged that underscores the importance and empiric basis of the *reorganization* step of the Marketing Mindset. This pattern of collaborations, partnerships, and joint ventures has been increasing, not so much in number as in magnitude, scope and variety. There are, on average, over three hundred significant healthcare mergers and acquisitions per year in the US. But even more than the numbers, it's the combinations and types of partnerships that are fascinating.

In the past, I understood healthcare mergers and acquisitions to be largely about gaining more market share through the combining of similar assets, commonly termed "horizontal mergers" (same local geography) or "market-extension mergers" (different geographies). In addition to the augmented market share and enlarged customer base, a potential advantage of these horizontal-type mergers is eliminating redundancies in and sharing the costs of fixed corporate business and administrative costs. Another obvious advantage is greater contract bargaining power between providers, payers, and suppliers.

While these horizontal and market extension mergers continue, I've observed an alternative partnership, the intent of which is to create synergistic, value-creating couplings of different assets and capabilities. This type of merger might be considered a "product-extension merger" in which companies who produce different but related products join together. One purpose of these product-extension merges is to enhance access to an enlarged and potentially new customer base, and therefore increase growth and market share. But these mergers go beyond market extension mergers by attempting to join complementary assets and offerings in ways that are more than merely additive.

From my perspective, these product-extension-like partnerships and ventures are a novel reorganization that can greatly enhance value from the customer perspective. I had not really understood their disruptive potential until I heard an executive from Walmart describe them. Marcus Osborne, the VP of health and wellness at Walmart, shared this comment during a recent interview I conducted with him: "The greatest disruption that will occur, will occur with entities who are savvy enough to understand that you can't do it alone... You have to have partners, and if you find those right kind of partners, and you bring the right kind of assets together, and resources, and the collective will, you can drive real change."[69]

Walmart has been testing the healthcare-delivery market for years, with numerous endeavors including their embedded walk-in clinics, their pharmacies and novel pharmacy pricing, and their retail healthcare-related products. They've also directly been testing their healthcare-delivery and reorganization capabilities in a significantly large internal venue. With over a million employees and an annual employee healthcare spend of over $4 billion, Walmart has been deploying and monitoring healthcare-delivery approaches and services within its own self-insured domain. It was fascinating to hear Marcus describe Walmart's intentions to enter healthcare delivery in a bolder, grander way than in the past; but what was even more fascinating was how they might potentially go about it. Marcus's message was clear—product-extending partnerships and reorganizations would be critical in the transformation of American healthcare and would likely play a significant role in Walmart's plan to expand its footprint in the healthcare-delivery market.

As I listened in awe to the picture that Marcus was painting, I began to think that if Walmart was strategizing that way, so must others—Amazon, Google, Apple, Microsoft, Target, CVS and Walgreens, along with the hundreds of smaller new-entrant healthcare companies and start-ups. I began to imagine what healthcare might look like if Amazon and Walmart decided to collaborate, or if IBM or Microsoft began to product-merge with retailers. One picture Marcus painted was that of a three product-extension merger. He described the combination of an in-store retailer (think Walmart) with a drive-by convenience retailer (think Chick-fil-A), combined with online digital retail and social-network customer experience (think Amazon).

During the course of our conversation, I began to imagine other product-extending combinations. What if Apple combined its cloud-based comprehensive health-record-keeping and biometric Apple-watch monitoring with the predictive analytics and consumer-relationship management of Salesforce? Or what if telecom companies like Comcast combined their evolving employee healthcare capabilities and services with the movie-making and entertainment capabilities of Netflix or Pixar?

Based on these types of conversations and similar observations, I've come to suspect that the next slew of major disruptions in healthcare may not arise from single entities. Instead, those disruptions may occur via multi-organizational product-extension mergers. Along with their collective synergistic product lines, these entities would bring with them a native, highly sophisticated understanding of consumer-centric, demand-side thinking and capabilities. Again, these types of partnerships will not just increase market share through the additive combination of similar assets. They will generate new value through innovative reorganization.

> *The next slew of major disruptions in healthcare may not arise from single entities. Instead, those disruptions may occur via multi-organizational product-extension mergers.*

CVS HEALTH/AETNA

One high-profile product-extension merger that is in progress at the time of this writing is the CVS/Aetna merger. CVS is the largest retail pharmacy chain in the country. There are over ten thousand stores and over one thousand Minute Clinics or retail-based clinics embedded in those stores. CVS also owns Caremark, which is one of the largest pharmacy-benefits managers (PBMs) in the country. So, the merged CVS/Aetna comprises the largest retail pharmacy chain, the largest PBM, one of the largest health-product retail chains, the largest chain of retail-based clinics, and now, with its approximately $60 billion acquisition of Aetna, one of the top three healthcare-insurance companies in the US. While size does play a role—their totaled annual revenue is estimated to be in the range of $250 billion—it's their newly combined synergistic capabilities that should allow them to enhance and develop products and services, as well as create savings (value) way beyond what their separate legacy systems might have accomplished.

But, the partnering doesn't end there. The situation is even more intricate and interesting because Aetna brings with it numerous value-enhancing joint ventures with provider groups. Aetna has already been actively developing joint health-insurance companies with hospital systems and provider groups.[70] It has also established numerous value-based joint ventures with pharmaceutical companies and device manufacturers. These mergers are more than simply the additive combination of assets. Aetna's goal was to create new value in healthcare by enabling provider groups, pharmaceutical companies, and device manufacturers to participate in contracts in which all stakeholders benefit from the lowering of costs and the elevation of health outcomes—each side bringing unique and synergistic capabilities to produce an extended-product-line approach. These fascinating and complex reorganizations reflect a merger-within-a-merger-type picture and represent yet another profound and empiric illustration of an emerging pattern of profound reorganizing disruptions in the healthcare market.

By merging with Aetna, CVS can begin to take financial or cost-of-care risk with the patients they serve. By having a health insurance arm, they now benefit from the cost savings they create and pass onto their customers and payers. This merger allows CVS to expand its portfolio as well as compete more effectively in a customer-oriented, value-based market. Additionally, given their well-established retail presence, the CVS/Aetna entity can cross-market and cross-sell insurance products, including Medicare Advantage.

By broadening its scope of assets and capabilities, CVS/Aetna's market capabilities will include:

1. value-based contracting for its partners,

2. health insurance for its corporate and individual customers,

3. medications for individual health consumers,

4. health-related products and durable medical equipment,

5. indirect medical care through its joint ventures, and

6. direct medical care in its minute clinics and stores.

With all these capabilities available to them, I wouldn't be surprised if CVS/Aetna began developing, supporting, and offering multiple segmented primary-care brands such as complex-chronic-care, condition-specific chronic disease management care, and even wellness-care brands, in addition to its already existing on-demand (Minute Clinic) brand.

While there is some concern that large mega-mergers such as CVS/Aetna will limit customer choice, I believe that quite the opposite will occur. Look—many consider this CVS acquisition to be a strategic response to what others are doing in the market such as Optum Health/United Health Group and Amazon. My point is that if CVS and Aetna are deploying these reorganizing strategies, so are others. That would mean that healthcare is evolving into an increasingly hypercompetitive market dominated by customer-oriented stakeholders. These stakeholders are all vying to continuously elevate their value proposition and differentiation to acquire and maintain their customer base. This puts the healthcare customer and consumer in a great position: increasing value, better customer service and experience, and expanded options. I would argue that the value proposition for the healthcare customer has never been better, and it will continue to improve.

OPTUM HEALTH VENTURES

CVS/Aetna is not an isolated case. In fact, as I just mentioned, some have opined that CVS may be a strategic response to the example of Optum/United Health Group (UHG). The two distinct businesses that make up UHG are United Health Care, one of the largest health insurance companies in the country, and OptumCare, a healthcare-service organization. UHG has a combined annual revenue of over $210 billion. The OptumCare division has three large sub-divisions that are separate but work together to support one another. The three divisions are: (1) a collection of clinical provider groups (Optum-Health); (2) a pharmacy-benefits manager (OptumRx), one of the three largest PBMs in the country; and (3) an analytics division (Optu-mInsight). OptumCare continues to very actively expand its provider base, accumulating primary-care and multi-specialty medical groups. At the time of this writing, it's in the process of acquiring Davita Medical Group. Once the Davita deal closes, Optum will employ or partner with nearly fifty thousand providers in primary and specialty care as well as urgent care. They've also begun to develop a surgical-care division as well. The market value and power of any one of these OptumCare divisions is stellar, but when combined, they're formidable. And when you add the insurance arm, UHG, it's one of the most impressive case studies and examples of value-enhancing reorganization unfolding in the US healthcare market.

The synergistic market capabilities created by Optum/UHG's evolving reorganization are myriad and complex. Through their insurance arm, they can assume financial risk for their healthcare customers, as well as for other provider groups. The PBM arm allows them to control and manage the costs and distribution of medications and medical devices. And the analytics arm gives them a major leg up on being able to understand how to identify customers who are at risk, optimally manage medical-care utilization, improve health outcomes, and minimize unnecessary and preventable medical expenditures. That analytic arm also provides them with customer intelligence that can create a more customized and engaging consumer experience. The reorganized entities within (Optum/UHG) create synergistic benefits in numerous ways—in an almost hedged-bet way. For example—on the volume-based side, they benefit by selling medications and clinical services; and on the value-based side, they benefit by driving costs down and outcomes up. So, similar to the CVS/Aetna reorganization, Optum/UHG has situated itself to perform well in the current volume-based, fee-for-service payment environment and in the emerging value-based, customer-oriented market. Optum/UHG will be competing with CVS/Aetna and numerous other entities out there that are also partnering, merging, morphing, and reorganizing. Far from limiting choice and convenience, or driving up costs, it is my impression that these new reorganizations are creating the potential for tremendous value-generation in the healthcare market. What we are witnessing is indeed a customer and consumer revolution in healthcare, and the reorganizing step of the Marketing Mindset is a major factor in facilitating that transformation.

> What we are witnessing is indeed a customer and consumer revolution in healthcare, and the reorganizing step of the Marketing Mindset is a major factor in facilitating that transformation.

THE "PAYVIDER" MOVEMENT

Healthcare-insurance companies and provider organizations are partnering to become "payviders," a hybrid of payer and provider. These so-called payviders are not new entities in healthcare delivery. They've existed for a while, but they were relatively scarce in the market. Kaiser is the quintessential example, but others exist, such as

Geisinger, Intermountain, and Sentara. The advantage of being a payvider is that in a cost-conscious, risk-based market, the combined insurer/provider entity benefits tremendously by producing cost savings. If your provider arm is highly efficient and cost-effective, your payer arm reaps the cost saving benefits, which can in return be used to further fund, grow, resource, and reward the provider arm. That's assuming, of course, that healthcare-customer experience and quality of care are an integral part of these organization's goals. And that seems to be the case if you look at real-life examples like Kaiser or Geisinger, which have been leaders and innovators for decades in producing cost-effective, high quality health outcomes and great customer experience. If payer and provider are separate—the predominant current construct—it's largely the payer who reaps the benefits of cost-effective care. The provider groups pour resources into being more efficient and cost-effective, but do not directly benefit from those savings and that value generation.

It requires tremendous resources—money, time, people, and planning—to create and maintain high-quality, safe, consumer-oriented, cost-effective healthcare. And, there are risks in reorganizing as a payvider. But the advantage, from a business/financial perspective, is that it more fully aligns and integrates the resource investment with the return on that investment. A provider that is not a payer does not fully realize the investment, because the cost savings goes to the payer. If you become your own payer, the returns directly accrue to you, or at least to your payer arm. This is the primary reason that payviders like Geisinger, Kaiser Permanente, and Intermountain Health have been so ahead of the curve in terms of developing cost-effective, high quality outcomes. They have an optimal structure for value-based care. What we're witnessing in the market—as evidenced by some of the examples I've shared—is, in part, a reorganizing movement toward an augmented product-extending payvider model. We'll see if this direction continues, but for now, it seems like it's picking up momentum.

In addition to the reorganizations described above, there are numerous collaborations and partnerships (reorganizations) in the employer (corporate) space that are disrupting the healthcare market with their promise to create and unleash greater value. First, we're seeing employers contracting directly with provider groups. Second, there are employer coalitions and joint ventures forming. And, third, we're seeing employers become highly active in recruiting and organizing vendors to optimize the healthcare of their employees. We'll discuss the first reorganization in the next chapter, but let's discuss the other two here.

EMPLOYER COALITIONS AND MERGERS

There are numerous employer coalitions and collaboratives that have emerged over the past few years—the Pacific Business Group on Health; the Northeast Business Group on Health; the National Business Group on Health; the Global Business Group on Health; the Global Chief Medical Officers Network of BUPA; the Health Enhancement Research Organization (HERO); the Integrated Benefits Institute; as well as employer coalitions facilitated by large consultancies such as Aon Hewitt, Mercer, Willis Towers Watson, Gallagher, and Buck Consulting, just to name a few. Although I typically avoid making predictions, I suspect that these coalitions and collaboratives will continue to expand and grow in importance, effectiveness, and influence. And new ones will appear, affording employers unprecedented market power and impact in terms of improved health outcomes and cost savings. We'll spend more time in chapter 10 discussing employer health activism and what might even be called an employer health revolution.

One watershed example of employer health activism and reorganization occurred in January 2018: the CEOs of Amazon, Berkshire Hathaway, and JPMorgan Chase announced that they were forming a separate joint-venture company to focus exclusively on improving health outcomes and experience, and reducing the costs of care for their employees. There was much fanfare in the news regarding the venture's focus on reducing administrative costs of care and potentially cutting out intermediaries such as pharmacy-benefits managers and insurers. There is no question that the announcement sent shock waves throughout the market—groundswells that have continued to trigger other significant shifts. Since that announcement, the language and posture of employers toward healthcare has shifted dramatically. But, even prior to this, in the couple of years leading up to it, Warren

Buffet, the CEO of Berkshire Hathaway, with his uniquely brilliant and premonitory flair, was vocally proclaiming that employers should not continue to accept low-value healthcare, which he asserted was undermining the financial well-being and profitability of American companies. His now well-known admonition to business leaders was and continues to be, "Healthcare costs are the hungry tapeworm of Corporate America." Much has been postulated in the news about the high likelihood that whatever solutions this joint venture comes up with, it won't be limited to their own employees. When they create a solution to lower their own employee health costs and improve outcomes, it's almost a given that they'll offer up those products and services to other employers and the healthcare market at large.

CLINICAL INTEGRATION NETWORKS

The reorganizations occurring in healthcare are not limited to insurance companies, employers, and retailers, they are also beginning to sweep through provider organizations. The "Clinical Integration Network," or CIN, is a legal entity that allows independent provider groups—hospitals and practices—to align and collaborate in an unprecedented way. The groups are allowed to refer and share a population of healthcare customers for which they've co-contracted. In the past, this sort of activity would have triggered anti-kickback laws. But, under the legal umbrella of the CIN, different provider entities can work closely together. There are, however, legal requirements, not the least of which is that this collective of hospital systems and provider groups must demonstrate and thoroughly document that they are collaborating jointly with the sole and explicit purpose of improving the clinical outcomes of care, improving efficiencies, and lowering avoidable costs.

As of 2015, there were over five hundred CIN's in the US, and the number is growing.[71] The partnering stakeholders which make up CIN's include large multi-hospital systems, individual hospitals, free-standing EDs, surgical centers, as well as independent primary-care, specialty, and multi-specialty practices. These partners collaborate in shared, value-based contracts to enhance value in various ways. They co-develop and adopt standardized protocols to enhance care. They set performance goals and monitor individual physicians against those goals. They set policies and incentives to foster physician engagement. They improve coordination of care between the stakeholder members. If their collective efforts deliver lower cost, high quality care, they do well financially. If they don't, there are no gains to be shared. As one might imagine, the coordination is complicated. It's hard enough to operate and manage a single clinical entity, but the challenges mount when a CIN's leadership attempts to align and organize multiple separate clinical groups. The jury is still out on whether or not this type of reorganization will deliver on the promise and whether a next-generation CIN-like approach will emerge. But, once again, it demonstrates that reorganizing is a critical component of the transition and transformation of healthcare delivery.

CROSSING SWIM LANES

I'd like to point out one aspect of this large, systemic, market-driven movement of healthcare organization. The examples provided demonstrate a blurring of traditional lines among legacy healthcare stakeholders and new entrant organizations. Health insurance companies, retailers, pharmacy chains, employers, dig-tech, and telecom companies, as well as start-ups, are explicitly crossing over into the provider swim lane. In the past, the narrative of this cross-over has been a bit more guarded and opaque—couched in statements like,

"We're here to support physicians and provider groups, to fill in the gaps, to augment the core services already being provided." But as the market reorganizations advance, the narrative is becoming far less hesitant and is taking a much more directly competitive stance. As Chris Holt, a leader in Amazon's Global Healthcare Division, put it, "We aren't trying to fit into any traditional definition of how things work in healthcare. We're trying to bring our own capabilities to the market. We've seen a tremendous willingness among our customer base to try out new things, even though they know that it might not be something they're used to. That's been very encouraging to us."[72]

In chapters 5 and 8, we described the market-driven movement that is underway—toward a hyper-segmented, interdependent rebranding of healthcare delivery. In chapter 9, we discussed how healthcare systems are reorganizing from healthcare to health systems and demonstrated the multiple ways in which *reorganizing* has become a critical transformational movement in healthcare delivery today, and is likely to remain one for years to come. Although "reorganizing" may not be as buzzworthy as revolutions in the digital, technological, and analytical realms, it may prove to be one of the most powerful healthcare innovations of our time.

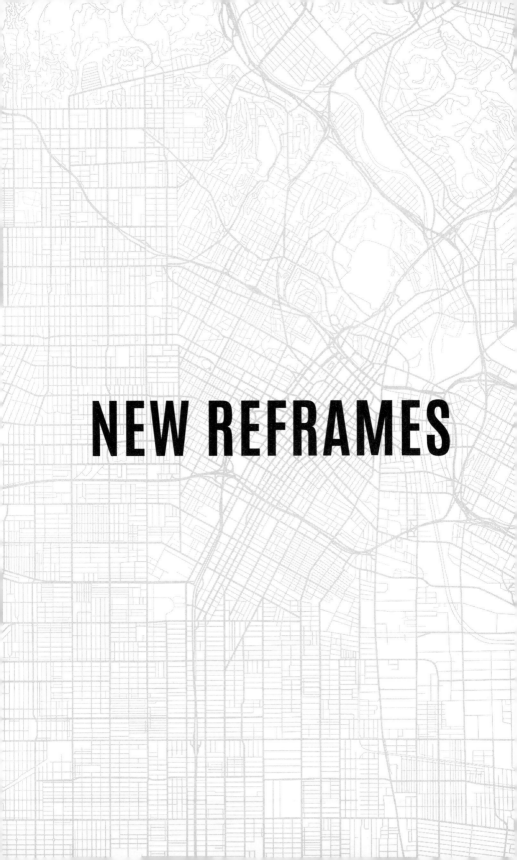

NEW REFRAMES

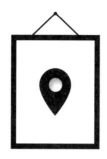

CHAPTER 10

GAME-CHANGING TRENDS

—It's tough to make predictions, especially about the future.

Yogi Berra

A colleague once shared with me his observation regarding emerging trends: they tend to happen with much greater certainty than we ascribe to them, but they tend to happen much later than we expect them to occur. I would agree that this has been true for emerging trends in the past. However, it appears to me that we're experiencing a marked acceleration of changes and disruptions in the healthcare market. So, I would not discount the possibility that game-changing healthcare trends will come much faster and much bigger than we have observed in the past few decades. In my presentations at conferences and board retreats, I refer to healthcare as being in a "phase-change" moment. In physics, a phase-change is that state between two different forms, like liquid and solid. Water at the freezing-point phase-change appears to be normal liquid water, but it's actually at the transition point of almost immediately becoming ice. What's important to note is that the phase-change occurs without any change in the chemical composition. It's simply a transfer of energy. And that is how I view our current moment in healthcare. On the surface, we appear to be in one phase, but we're actually at that rapid energy transitioning point of converting into a very different state.

There is one point that's important to emphasize at the start of this chapter on trends and transitions. Nothing in this book is based on predictions about the future. The fundamental reframes and shifts I've described in this book are derived and distilled from observed realities in the market. A corollary point is that the many mega-trends touched upon in this book and this chapter are not isolated events. Instead, they are, from my perspective, manifestations of the larger context of the Marketing Mindset. Therefore, this affords one the ability to use the Marketing Mindset as a framework from which to contextualize and better understand any given trend, strategy, or tactic, and to provide greater perspective on how to respond strategically and proactively to market forces in general.

The following is a list of game-changing trends that have been mentioned in this book—some more explicitly than others. This is not a comprehensive list nor a prioritized one, and you may recognize that there is both overlap and nuanced relationships among the trends.

Game-changing trends in healthcare today include:

- digital healthcare

- behavior design

- predictive analytics and artificial intelligence

- retail medicine

- employer health activism

- well-being and human performance

- personalized precision medicine

- consumerism

- transparency (cost, quality, outcomes, and experience)

- risk-based contracts

- prepaid and capitated payment models

- innovative partnerships, collaborations, and joint ventures

- payvider organizations

Since this is not a book about healthcare trends but about the significant underlying reframes, forces, and factors that are driving them, the goal of this chapter will not be to fill in the gaps in our understanding of all the above-mentioned trends. Instead, I'll focus on two of them: digital healthcare and employer health activism. The reasons for selecting these two specific trends to expand upon are two-fold. First, they represent immensely powerful and proximal (in full swing) market-shifting forces that are of immediate importance. Second, they're highly generative; that is, they are driving and facilitating many of the other trends. As you'll see, I'll spend less time on "digital healthcare" because there is already so much focus and awareness of it.

Digital Healthcare

The redesign of healthcare is actively being deployed through digital, virtual, and in-person processes. The invitation "call, click, or come in" is one we're increasingly hearing in systems across the country, and it exemplifies the emerging multi-media and multi-channel makeup of healthcare. While in-person healthcare will almost certainly continue to be a mainstay for the near future, it's already well understood and accepted that, conservatively speaking, anywhere between 25 to 50 percent of ambulatory (non-hospital) visits can be virtual, digital, and asynchronous. An editorial piece published in an October 2017 issue of *The Annals of Internal Medicine* reimagines the in-person visit of the future as what we will consider "tertiary" or highly-specialized care.[73] If one pushes this concept further, it really makes me wonder whether "visits"—as we understand them today—will exist at all in the future of healthcare, especially with the technologic capabilities of 24/7 monitoring and analytics, coupled with automated algorithmic, machine-generated responses. Keep in mind that digital, virtual, and in-person human interactive modalities are not mutually exclusive. Livongo is a wonderful example of a seamless hybrid of modalities for type 2 diabetes that leverages cutting-edge digital care, machine learning, and automated responses but also relies on traditional telephonic and in-person visits as well.[74] Virta—a fully virtual diabetes clinic that I serve as an industry advisor for—is a brilliant and effective example of an almost exclusive reliance on asynchronous digital care for type 2 diabetes.[75] Both are demonstrating remarkable outcomes as well as superior customer experience with a reduction in overall costs of care.[76]

> *It really makes me wonder whether "visits"—as we understand them today—will exist at all in the future of healthcare.*

Many misconstrue the digital redesign of healthcare delivery as some sort of broad-stroke panacea—a way to right the inadequacies of the legacy approach. This is a misguided perspective. Digital delivery, in and of itself, does not guarantee a customer-oriented approach. It does not guarantee consumer adoption or cost-effectiveness. As Kevan Mabbutt of Intermountain Health has said, "... using digital platforms, analytics, and engagement to help support, navigate, inform—and to some extent even deliver—care, is definitely a part of what we're talking about here. But, it's not the same thing as being consumerist. It's often just a means to it."[77] Mabbutt's opinion is substantiated by the research on the effectiveness of wearable digital devices in improving healthful behaviors and outcomes. An article in the *Journal of the American Medical Association* concluded, "Although wearable devices have the potential to facilitate health behavior change, this change might not be driven by these devices alone. Instead, the successful use and potential health benefits related to these devices depends more on the design of the engagement strategies than on the features of their technology. Ultimately, it is the engagement strategies—the combinations of individual encouragement, social competition and collaboration, and effective feedback loops—that connect with human behavior."[78]

In and of itself, digital technology does not reframe healthcare. If anything, the digital platform requires an even greater adherence to the demand-side, consumer-oriented principles of the Marketing Mindset. One reason for this is that digital is still a relatively new channel for engagement. It requires

> *In and of itself, digital technology does not reframe healthcare. If anything, the digital platform requires an even greater adherence to the demand-side, consumer-oriented principles of the Marketing Mindset.*

what Silicon Valley entrepreneurs refer to as a "10x experience." In other words, digital applications and interfaces don't just need to be as good as their non-virtual analogues; they need to be much better in order to attract, engage, and compete for customers in a sustained way. Digital apps and platforms require a much greater adherence to the principles of good design, in large part because there is little-to-no human factor to fill in the gaps.

Utilizing digital channels successfully will require rigorous adherence to the Marketing Mindset. Of the thousands of new healthcare-related digital applications put on the market, the overwhelming majority do not deliver on a sustained value proposition. Some interpret this outcome to mean that digital doesn't work. Quite the opposite, digital healthcare delivery can work as well as, if not better than, non-digital, *if* its creators follow the mindset of rebranding, redesigning, and reorganizing. Without a keen awareness of what digital is and isn't, as well as an understanding of the behavioral and design principles that actually create the healthful changes and consumer-centric outcomes we're attempting to achieve, we could spend years going down a path that brings us no closer to our customers and their desired outcomes.

On the other hand, if designed well, digital and virtual platforms represent an unprecedented enabler for healthcare delivery. Sean Duffy, CEO of Omada Health, refers to digital as another "ether moment" in healthcare. During one of our interviews together, Sean reminded me of the introduction of ether in the surgical suite and how that transformed the field of surgery. Prior to ether, surgical procedures were greatly limited. Patients could not be put to sleep or anesthetized, so surgical procedures had to be performed quickly, *very* quickly, as people were forcibly being held down. The introduction of ether allowed surgery to be conducted under a very different set of circumstances and opened up the opportunity for the lengthy and complex life-saving surgical procedures that exist today. The analogy has merit. Ether led to the anesthesia platform that unleashed, enabled, and amplified the potential of surgical care. In a similar vein, digital already has and will continue to unleash, enable, and amplify the value proposition and immense potential currently locked in our healthcare-delivery system. Picking up on Sean's insightful analogy, I would suggest that digital represents a "beyond-ether" moment, in that the innovation of ether was still limited by its in-person deployment. Digital health innovation, on the other hand, is a networked phenomenon that exists in a completely virtual, analytically enabled environment. It's more like the "ether-moment-on-steroids." If branded, designed, and organized well, digital healthcare can facilitate a value proposition, an experience, and outcomes that far exceed what we've been able to accomplish within the limitations of our current in-person or telephonic encounters. Let's briefly explore this issue.

AUTOMATED MONITORING, TRACKING, AND MEASUREMENT

In the past, if you wanted to have your physician, nurse, or any other provider assess some biometric—such as blood pressure, temperature, or blood-glucose level—that process typically required an in-person visit. With digital technologies, biometrics can be tracked automatically and even continuously—weekly, daily, hourly, or by the second. Beyond tracking, that data can now be monitored, analyzed, and even responded to automatically, as well as asynchronously. Machine-learning algorithms can identify—in real time—patterns that no human mind could. They can predict rising risks—again, in real time—or the worsening of chronic conditions;

thereby allowing for immediate intervention and the prevention of outcomes such as emergency-room visits, hospitalizations, acute events with morbid outcomes, and higher costs. Digital monitoring and machine-generated responses don't require an individual to wait for his or her next office visit to be assessed and treated. It's added a whole new dimension to preventive medical care and chronic disease management.

PROACTIVE AND EFFECTIVE
INTERVENTIONS AND ENGAGEMENT

All the behavior-design techniques and tools at our disposal today—like gamification, triggers, social connectivity, and behavioral-economic nudges—can be programmed into a digital healthcare-delivery platform. Far from restricting our activities or manipulating our behaviors, these tools make it easier and more convenient for us to take the more healthful course of behavior. As we know from the literature, small directed healthful habits send us off on larger and sustained positive trajectories. And as these behaviorally designed, neuropsychologic-based software programs guide our behaviors, they also monitor our behaviors and learn our proclivities and dislikes. Numerous consumer-response tests are programmed into the digital platforms we use daily (Facebook, Google, Amazon), and the output of that accumulated testing is a responsive software that becomes increasingly more customized and personalized.

One universal goal of dig/tech gurus and innovators is to design a digital experience that is so relevant, engaging, and customized that it almost feels like it was custom-made specifically for each individual. Glen Tullman, the founder and executive chairman of Livongo, shared a quote with me by Arthur C. Clarke (the noted science fiction writer and futurist): "Technology perfectly applied is indistinguishable from magic." Digital innovators have already begun to explore the infinite potential to deliver on this magic. As we discovered in our discussion on design principles in chapter 7, it's not enough to be clinically relevant. The experience must continue to captivate the user in novel ways. The point for leaders to remember is that digital is neither a strategy nor a design, but a tool that can greatly amplify both. My message to healthcare leaders is that our goal should not be to digitize healthcare, but to humanize it.

> *Our goal should not be to digitize healthcare, but to humanize it.*

Employer Health Activism[79]

In chapter 9, we touched upon the notion that employers are a powerful player in the healthcare market. In my estimation, employers are *the* most powerful force for change in the healthcare market today. They have been the *sleeping giants of the US healthcare market* for years, but now they're awake, active, and perhaps a bit angry.

Let me provide a bit of "employer health" backstory.

Employers have, for years, experienced healthcare costs as one of their major expenses and one

> *Employers have been the sleeping giants of the US healthcare market for years, but now they're awake, active, and perhaps a bit angry.*

that continues to rise each year, greatly out of proportion to CDI and other market benchmarks. At the time of this writing, it appears that the rise in employer healthcare costs is going to increase this following year by about 5 percent. A great resource for understanding the healthcare concerns of employers and employees is the University of Utah Health Survey—a multi-year survey of hundreds of employers that exposes some surprising statistics. For example, the survey reveals that less than 50 percent of employees believe their out-of-pocket healthcare costs are affordable; and only about 50 percent of employers believe that healthcare costs are affordable or that their employees have access to high-quality providers.[80]

As you might imagine, there have been extensive and intensive efforts to understand those costs better. The employer "health-benefits-advisory" industry has deployed numerous maneuvers to control those costs—from health risk assessments, to wellness coaching, to care management and chronic-disease case management, to preventive campaigns around weight loss and smoking cessation. A recent trend has been the deployment of High Deductible Health Plans (HDHP) in which employees are responsible for the first few thousand dollars of healthcare costs each year (out-of-pocket). The HDHP movement had swelled to the point that nearly 40 percent of corporations had adopted it. However, some statistics recently indicate that the industry might be backpedaling. For the first time in six years, according to a report by the National Business Group on Health, 2018 witnessed a 9 percent decrease in HDHPs.[81] I suspect the percentage of employers utilizing HDHP's will continue to plummet.[82]

Merely shifting healthcare costs from employer to employee did not do anything to resolve the underlying ineffectiveness and inefficiencies.

There are numerous reasons for the failure of the HDHP experiment, the major one being that merely shifting healthcare costs from employer to employee did not do anything to resolve the underlying ineffectiveness and inefficiencies of the healthcare-delivery system. Zack Cooper, a healthcare economist and policy expert at Yale, along with his colleagues, demonstrated that within the current construct, employees don't have the resources to make healthful and cost-effective decisions about healthcare utilization.[83] Healthcare-benefits advisors, like David Contorno of Health Rosetta, go even further to argue, with good evidence, that it's ridiculous to assume that any individual employee can comprehend the complexities of the opaque healthcare system. In fact, Contorno points out that while HDHPs will lower costs in the short run by decreasing utilization across the board, it also reduces appropriate utilization leading to rebound costs, frustrated employees, and unintended consequences from misguided healthcare decision-making.[84] There are companies out there offering some guidance on cost and quality; but, to date, that information has been disappointing. So, the position of groups like Health Rosetta is that, at least for the present moment, it is the responsibility and duty of employers and their health-benefits advisors to set up a value-based benefits and healthcare-delivery program that assists and guides employees to make cost-effective, outcomes-oriented decisions—decisions that are in the best interest of the employees and their families.

Unsustainable costs and a lack of demonstrably effective outcomes are the major reasons for why employers have risen to be the prime force of disruption in healthcare today.[85] Also note that the direct medical costs of employee health are compounded by a factor of 2 or 3 due to the costs of absenteeism and lost productivity resulting from illness and or medical treatment. Employers—non-healthcare corporations—are also realizing that if they can develop a product or service that successfully, sustainably, and safely lowers the cost of care, they have the opportunity to enter into and disrupt the $3.4 trillion healthcare industry that comprises nearly 20 percent of the US GDP. They are beginning to realize that if they can reduce even a fraction of the gross inefficiencies and ineffectiveness, there's a huge opportunity for value and revenue generation. Given the internal and external opportunities, employers are no longer waiting for legacy healthcare stakeholders to make needed change in health-care delivery. They are, without question, *reframing and redefining* the system. As you'll see in the examples that follow, employers are applying a Marketing Mindset to healthcare, and are *rebranding, redesigning,* and *reorganizing* healthcare delivery.

THE "DIRECT-TO-EMPLOYER" MOVEMENT

An August 2018 article in the *Wall Street Journal* described a "Health-Care Deal" that General Motors struck with the Henry Ford Health System in Detroit, Michigan.[86] The General Motors deal is not an isolated disruptive partnership but part of a larger national movement to cut coverage costs and improve care quality. The article references a National Business Group on Health (NBGH) survey of over 170 large employers, which indicated that 11 percent of employers say they plan to engage in similar large-scale, direct-contract deals with healthcare providers in the coming year.[87] To further corroborate this, the Willis Towers Watson 2017 "Best Practices in Health Care Employer Survey" of nearly seven hundred employers discovered that over 90 percent of the employers surveyed were "aggressively" moni-toring their vendor partners and actively seeking high-performing provider networks.[88]

This direct-to-employer movement is a result of employers realizing that they must assume responsibility for directing their employees' healthcare as well as more closely measuring and moni-toring its demonstrated value. Employers are seeking ways to prevent high-cost crises and are looking for ways to prevent the downstream costs and morbidity of chronic health conditions. They're looking for ways to drive appropriate behaviors such as preventive primary care; and to discourage costly and potentially harmful behaviors such as inappropriate utilization of high-cost diagnostics, ED visits, and many common surgical procedures. The bottom line is that employers are looking for ways to

Employers are looking for ways to design their health benefits and health offerings based on value, not on volume.

design their health benefits and health offerings based on value, not on volume.

Comcast has 225,000 employees and dependents with an annual healthcare spend of approximately $1.3 billion. Instead of going the route of high-deductible health plans, the company is supporting its employees in navigating healthcare and in making prudent decisions. Comcast has independently invested in and directly contracted with healthcare vendors to assist them with reorganizing and redirecting not just health-benefits design, but the actual delivery of care.[89] Some of the vendors include: *Accolade*, which supplies healthcare navigators; *Grand Rounds*, which provides expert second opinions for high-cost, highly invasive surgical procedures; *Doctor on Demand,* which supplies telehealth virtual visits with clinicians; and *Brightside,* which provides financial-wellness coaching.

THE "CENTERS-OF-EXCELLENCE" MOVEMENT

Employer-based healthcare claims and quality data reveals that there are nationally recognized medical centers with world-class outcomes in certain high-cost, high-volume specialized procedures and treatments. These specialties include orthopedic and neurosurgery, oncology chemotherapy and treatment, and invasive cardiology procedures and surgery. National employers like Walmart, Lowe's, as well as many others, contract either directly or indirectly with these "Centers of Excellence" (COE). Up until now, employees have been given a choice about whether or not to seek out a second opinion, but it appears that, in the future, second opinions will be required. Many employers currently nudge their employees by reducing or eliminating the cost of treatments if employees avail themselves of the Centers of Excellence when seeking a second opinion. The Willis Towers Watson annual healthcare employer survey showed that by 2019, 77 percent of employers plan to use COEs within their health plans, and 21 percent plan to use them through a "carve-out" provider.[90]

One might suppose that employers are negotiating and contracting with these COEs for lower costs on a per-procedure basis. But as I've recently discovered, that's not the primary cost-saving mechanism driving employers to partner with COEs. Now, it is generally the case that the clinical outcomes of the COE surgeries and treatments are superior—with fewer complications, fewer hospital readmissions, and faster recovery times; and all these factors lead to better outcomes and an overall reduction in costs. But the overwhelming cost savings and larger value proposition is actually due to a reduction in inappropriate overutilization.

As Marcus Osborne, Walmart's VP of health and wellness, put it at the 2018 HLTH conference, "what we've learned is that it matters more to assess a provider on *appropriateness of utilization* than it does on quality, because you can game quality by doing inappropriate things!"[91] The experience of employers like Walmart exposes the fact that a significant percentage of referred specialty treatments and surgical procedures are revealed to be unnecessary and even harmful.

When an employee is referred to a COE, that second opinion begins with an assessment of the validity of the diagnosis, and the clinical appropriateness of the procedure. The results are shocking and disturbing. According to Walmart, there is a staggering percentage of reversals in diagnosis and proposed treatments as a result of these second-opinion COE evaluations. For example, 25 to 50 percent of all initially recommended surgeries are overturned! Over 50 percent of planned spine surgeries are overturned! Over 80 percent of initially proposed intracardiac stent placements are overturned! Over 10 percent of all cancer diagnoses are found to be blatantly wrong! And over 50 percent of all initial cancer treatment recommendations are revised! Walmart's experience is mirrored in the medical literature. The Mayo Clinic, for example, published a 2018 study demonstrating that of nearly three hundred specialty referrals from primary-care doctors, over one-fifth of the diagnoses were wrong, and nearly two-thirds of the diagnoses or treatments had to be modified. [92]

It's important to note that unnecessary procedures are not without risk and morbidity. Recovery time can be weeks, if not months, especially if there is a complication. Sadly, some employees never make it back to work at all—a devastating outcome for individuals and their families—and especially tragic when the procedure wasn't indicated in the first place. In other words, the total costs to employers and employees go far beyond the immediate costs of the surgery or treatment. As I mentioned previously, it's been estimated that two-thirds of total healthcare costs are due to productivity loss—people being out of work or at work, but less productive. By appropriately overturning

Centers of Excellence are helping employees and employers avoid potentially dangerous complications and outcomes.

unnecessary procedures and treatments, second-opinion COEs are helping employees and employers avoid potentially dangerous complications and outcomes, as well as the pain, time, and costs of recovery.

According to Osborne, the savings from these COE second opinions amounts to over $1 billion annually for Walmart, which represents a significant percentage, given their approximately $4 billion annual total healthcare spend.

For those concerned that this could become a systematic way of denying necessary surgeries and procedures, that's unlikely for at least the following reasons:

- When the subspecialty COEs overturn initial recommendations, they turn down the potential opportunity to perform the surgery or provide treatment, and therefore turn down the revenue opportunity.

- The overwhelming bias in our healthcare system is toward overutilization. We know that medical overutilization makes up approximately 40 percent of the over $1 trillion in wasteful (and harmful) healthcare spending in our country. With that amount of potential revenue at stake, it's easy to see how the bias in the industry is to over-diagnose and overtreat. Healthcare consumers are biased toward overutilization as well. In many ways, it's easier to get a knee replacement or spine disc procedure than it is to make a series of slow-to-result lifestyle changes like eating healthier, exercising more, and losing weight.

OTHER EMPLOYER MOVEMENTS

Somewhere between 30 percent to 50 percent of all employee ED visits are, in fact, non-emergent and/or preventable. Initiatives to address this, such as on-site clinics, near-site clinics, and urgent-care centers are being deployed by employers across the country. In 2018, one-third of employers with over five thousand employees offered on-site medical care, with another 11 percent planning to launch them in 2019.[93] These interventions not only prevent costly and unnecessary ED visits, they also allow employees convenient access to primary preventive and acute care without having to take significant time off from work.

Medication pricing is another major cost driver for employees, and represents one of the most significant and increasing line items not only for employers, but for healthcare in general. Employers are beginning to take this matter into their own hands by changing how they pay for their employees' pharmaceutical costs. They are now looking for value-based pharmacy-benefits managers outside of the mainstream legacy-player market. Some are engaging with or even forming coalitions to bargain directly with pharmaceutical companies for lower and more affordable drug pricing.

Employer health activism is clearly data-driven. Employers are using highly sophisticated analytic and actuarial tools to identify which conditions are impacting their employees' health in terms of direct medical costs and the indirect costs of lost productivity. With the support of large, national consulting firms, they have become increasingly aware of the specific cost impact of acute and chronic conditions such as stroke, heart attacks, diabetes, obesity, asthma, migraines, back and joint degeneration, depression, and even stress, as well as the impact of unhealthful habits such as cigarette smoking and lack of exercise.

Below is a list of some of the employer-based healthcare solutions that demonstrate how much and how specifically employers are addressing their organizations' healthcare needs.

CHECKLIST OF EMPLOYER-BASED HEALTHCARE BENEFIT SOLUTIONS

ADOPT:

- ✓ direct primary care (prepaid/capitated, open primary care network)
- ✓ value-based pharmacy plan design and pricing alternatives
- ✓ "second-opinion" centers-of-excellence
- ✓ transparent broker/advisor relationships
- ✓ high-performance (value-based) benefits plan design

ENCOURAGE AND INCENTIVIZE:

- ✓ utilization of primary preventive care and convenient urgent care
- ✓ value-based, lower-cost options
- ✓ digital enablement of consumer-oriented services and information
- ✓ innovative, condition-specific offerings and services

OFFER (AT LOW OR NO COST):

- ✓ convenient access to primary care and urgent care
- ✓ virtual primary care using telehealth

✓ navigators to coach and guide customers regarding options and utilization

✓ shared decision-making tools to reduce inappropriate utilization

✓ 24-hour hotline

✓ wellness and well-being programs

REDUCE OR ELIMINATE:

✓ co-pays (and any other costs) for primary and preventive care

✓ co-pays (and any other costs) for chronic-disease management

✓ unnecessary testing and diagnostics

✓ unnecessary specialty referrals

✓ inappropriate and unnecessary emergency-room visits

STANDARDIZE AND FOCUS ON:

✓ proven chronic-disease-management protocols of care

✓ social determinants of health and behavioral-health interventions

✓ high-tech, high-cost conditions such as oncology, cardiology, musculoskeletal injuries, and high-risk maternity

✓ complex-case management

This list of these employer-based solutions, and the many other emergent options to come, are important for employees and employers, and especially for corporate HR benefits managers. But these initiatives are insufficient. They won't achieve optimal outcomes unless they're utilized in a comprehensive framework such as the Marketing Mindset:

1. A *rebranded, value-based approach to payment*: The payment to benefits advisors, third-party administrators, or insurers must be aligned with employee/employer health cost-savings. If these entities' revenues are tied to increased premiums or higher employee health costs, a perverse incentive exists which can prevent true value-based care.

2. *Redesigned health benefits*: Optimally, employers should be designing benefits to assist and nudge employees to make healthful decisions for themselves and their families. Employers must recognize and support the priorities from the employee perspective, not from the perspective of the HR benefits manager, benefits advisor, third-party administrator, or insurer.

3. *Reorganized benefits structure*: Employers, benefit advisors, and insurers must align themselves with providers and provider groups that optimize care through appropriate utilization, outstanding quality, and excellent customer service, including access to appropriate care.

COALITIONS AND NETWORKS SUPPORTING THE EMPLOYER HEALTH-ACTIVIST MOVEMENT

I suspect that employer coalitions and networks emerging in the market over the next couple of years will incorporate, expand upon, standardize, and scale these and other employer-based healthcare initiatives in unprecedented ways. I strongly suspect that US healthcare will become much more employer-directed than in the past.

There are numerous coalitions supporting employers that already exist and are gaining momentum. Regional, national, and international groups such as the Pacific Business Group on Health (PBGH), the National Business Group on Health (NBGH), the Global Business Group on Health (GBGH), and the Health Enhancement Research Organization (HERO) have amassed hundreds of high-profile corporate member organizations that come together to share, vet, and curate best practices in improving employee health and well-being. In addition to the initiatives we've already discussed, these coalitions of human resource executives, benefits managers, wellness officers, medical personnel, and researchers focus their efforts on creating a culture of health and wellness within corporations. Their initiatives are supported by a growing body of evidence that correlates overall health and wellness with improvements in engagement, loyalty, lower absenteeism and presenteeism, and fewer disability claims, as well as with enhanced customer service and other markers of organizational performance. Brian Marcotte, the CEO of the NBGH and GBGH summarizes the movements' intention: "Employers would like to cover more value-based services and provide a higher level of coverage ... whether it's chronic condition management or preventative services or centers of excellence, there is a real opportunity to get back into design based on value."[94]

Earlier, I mentioned Health Rosetta, founded by David Chase and Sean Schantzen. Its mission is: to identify value-based practices that are clinically effective and cost-effective, and to directly train benefits advisors and managers to deploy these practices.[95] Health Rosetta has outlined several critical employee-health-benefit elements—a "blueprint for high-performance," which are well worth learning about.[96] To date, the Health Rosetta group has brought a few hundred benefits advisors into their membership, all while maintaining a strict entrance criterion. They've worked with dozens of employers and are rapidly gaining recognition for the health outcomes and savings they produce. The Health Rosetta approach is refreshingly customer-oriented and employee-centered. Their primary focus is on doing the right things for employees. They advocate for eliminating employees' costs of primary preventive care and basic chronic disease management; and go so far as to advocate for eliminating the costs of surgical procedures such as hip replacements, in conjunction with contracting with value-based providers.[97] The financials work out well for both employers and employees.

Health Rosetta's goal is to assist employers in side-stepping the traditional, predominant fee-for-service, volume-incentivized healthcare-delivery system. Chase points to three core reasons he believes employers are going to be a "highly disruptive force" in the coming years: (1) employers can act much more swiftly than federal and state policymakers, and faster than traditional healthcare providers; (2) mid- and large-sized companies understand the ROI of investing in R&D and are more open to investing in innovation than legacy healthcare organizations; and (3) new-entrant entrepreneurs can be sponsored by and collaborate with employers much more easily than attempting to work within the constraints of hospital systems. I would add to Chase's list the opportunity for these employers to enter into the $3.5 trillion healthcare delivery market as a vendor or even as a provider.

A Final Word on Game-Changing Trends

I've chosen to focus on two mega-trends in healthcare because I believe them to be most immediately relevant to overall impact and broad outcomes in the market. The sleeping giant of employer-based healthcare has only just begun to awaken and stir, and the same could be said of the digital and analytics healthcare revolution. What makes these mega-trends even more disruptive is that the most competitive stakeholders deploying them are doing so within the context of the Marketing Mindset reframe.

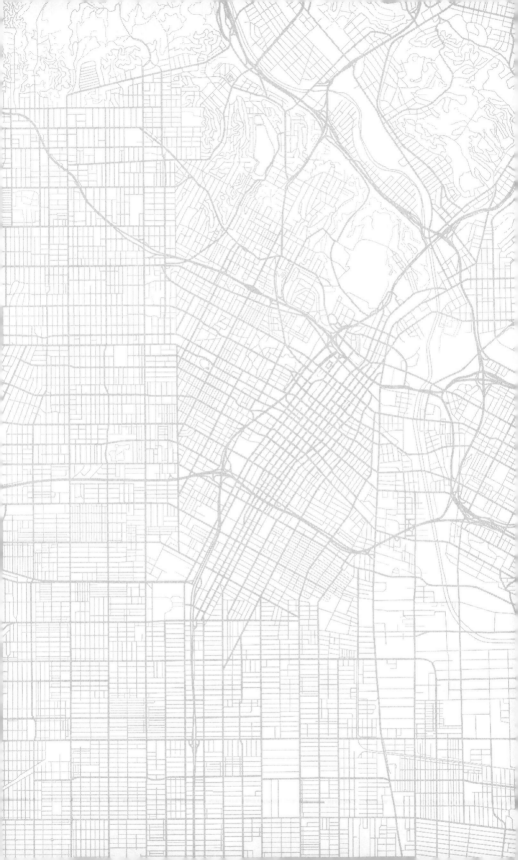

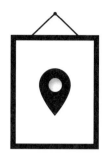

CHAPTER 11

THE "SOCIAL DETERMINANTS OF HEALTH" REFRAME

Social determinants of health is an abstract term; but for millions of Americans, it is a very tangible, frightening challenge: How can someone manage diabetes if they are constantly worrying about how they're going to afford their meals each week? How can a mother with an asthmatic son really improve his health if it's their living environment that's driving his condition? This can feel like a frustrating, almost fruitless position for a healthcare provider, who understands what is driving the health conditions they're trying to treat, who wants to help, but can't simply write a prescription for healthy meals, a new home, or clean air."

—Alex Azar, secretary of Health & Human Services[98]

Digital healthcare and employer health activism are integral to the transformation of healthcare today. It would be negligent not to consider them in any strategic planning discussion. Another critical consideration is how to weave the Social Determinants of Health (SDOH) into any strategic healthcare reframe discussion.

Background

In September of 2007 a colleague emailed me an article from the *New England Journal of Medicine* (NEJM) entitled "We Can Do Better — Improving the Health of the American People."[99] He told me the article provided epidemiologic and scientific support for what I had been speaking about for years in terms of better understanding the context of care for our patients. He thought it might help us better understand and focus our efforts. I was so struck by the article that I began including its data and graphics in most of my presentations.

The article, by Steven Schroeder, MD, provided a summation of a larger body of research literature demonstrating that what determined health morbidity and premature death, for the most part, was not a lack of medical care, but instead, social, environmental, and behavioral causes. More specifically, the breakdown was 40 percent due to "behavioral patterns," 15 percent directly due to "social causes," 5 percent due to "environmental exposures," 30 percent due to "genetic predispositions," and only 10 percent due to a lack of "healthcare." So, according to this and other data, approximately 60 percent of our health outcomes are determined by social causes while only 10 to 20 percent are due to what we consider our healthcare-delivery system. Put another way, if you add

Approximately 60 percent of our health outcomes are determined by social causes while only 10 to 20 percent are due to what we consider our healthcare delivery system.

up all the impact of diagnostic testing, medications, surgical procedures, and other medical interventions, that only amounts to a 10 percent impact in our health outcomes in the US. It's a staggering statistic with implications that should shake the very foundations of our approach to healthcare in this country and across the globe.

The National Academy of Medicine and the World Health Organization both recognize the validity of the science and epidemiologic evidence supporting a SDOH reframe. It's further supported, as we discussed back in chapter 1, by the observation that other developed nations across the globe achieve far superior health and longevity outcomes than we do in the US. And they do this by spending far less on clinical care and much more on the social determinants of health that impact individuals' behaviors and living circumstances. So, what are these so-called "social determinants of health?"

While this is not an exhaustive list, the social determinants of health include: poverty, unemployment, inadequate housing and unsafe neighborhoods, lack of healthful foods, lack of transportation, lack of education, the inability to be upwardly mobile and break transgenerational poverty, substance abuse and dependence, violence, social isolation and loneliness, the disruption or destruction of communities and social infrastructures, and a lack of meaning and purpose in one's life. A clever phrase that sums up the impact of the SDOH is, *one's zip code is a better predictor of health and longevity than one's genetic code*. Let's look at some data that supports this claim.

One's zip code is a better predictor of health and longevity than one's genetic code.

HEALTH PRIORITIZATION PROTOCOL

ACUTE INTERVENTIONAL CARE
Tertiary and Quaternary Care

CHRONIC DISEASE MANAGEMENT
Secondary Care

CLINICAL PRIMARY PREVENTION
Routine clinical care

WELLNESS
Care of physical health

WELLBEING
Care of social & emotional needs

SOCIETAL INFRASTRUCTURE
Care of community

Dr. Richard Cooper's 2016 book, entitled *Poverty and the Myths of Health Care Reform*, draws on decades of research to demonstrate that high-cost healthcare utilization (i.e., ED visits and hospitalizations) is inversely proportional to income level, while poor health outcomes are directly proportional to low incomes.[100] That is, the poorer you are, the more likely you are to utilize EDs and hospitals, and the less likely you are to have good overall health outcomes.

A 2016 study published in the *Journal of the American Medical Association* found that the top 5 percent of income earners in the US gained almost three years of life expectancy since 2001, while the bottom 5 percent made no real gains. Health improvement in older adults has been concentrated among white, well-educated, and higher-income individuals; older racial/ethnic minorities, those less educated, and lower-income individuals have experienced declining health.[101] Another study from July 2017 in the *Journal of the American Medical Association* demonstrated growing disparities in health and longevity in the US. The researchers concluded, "Much of the variation in life expectancy between counties can be explained by a combination of socioeconomic and race/ethnicity factors, behavioral and metabolic risk factors, and health care factors. Policy action targeting socioeconomic factors and behavioral and metabolic risk factors may help reverse the trend of increasing disparities in life expectancy in the United States."[102] The authors stated that the difference in life expectancy between disparate counties and zip codes in the US can be as much as twenty years![103]

There are numerous other studies and a significant body of research that we could review and cite. But the bottom line here is that tremendous inequities exist in healthcare and in health outcomes—disparities which degrade our children, our families, our communities, our society, and our country. While we pour tremendous resources and effort into solving these problems through traditional medical/clinical intervention, the literature is clear that social and behavioral factors play, by far, the biggest role in determining our healthcare utilization, healthcare costs, and health outcomes.[104] We, as a nation, need a more explicit, standardized, and systematic way to prioritize our attention, our strategies, and our resources on the SDOH.

> We, as a nation, need a more explicit, standardized, and systematic way to prioritize our attention, our strategies, and our resources on the social determinants of health.

The Healthcare Prioritization Protocol

Despite encouraging examples of health systems that clearly understand the value of the SDOH in reframing healthcare, it seems that the SDOH still remains a relatively low priority on a national scale. We continue to pour the overwhelming majority of our health-related resources—at the institutional, local, and national levels—into clinical approaches, even though the SDOH has been shown to have the overwhelming impact on health outcomes.[105] The reasons are both simple and complex, but they do reveal and signal the need for a fundamental healthcare-system *redesign* and *reorganization*. Our legacy healthcare system is simply not designed or organized to take care of the SDOH or to optimally enhance health in this way.

What is required is a system-wide reframe—a reorienting, redefining, and redirecting of strategies, tactics, and resources. What we need in order to expand and spread this SDOH reframe movement is to have a standardized, prioritized approach.

Toward this end, I've crafted a reframe protocol called the Healthcare Prioritization Protocol (HPP). Its purpose is to support leaders in operationalizing the SDOH reframe more fully and seamlessly into the larger, extended healthcare-delivery domain. It is a high-level guide to the prioritization, adoption, and implementation of solutions targeting the SDOH. Forward-thinking institutions and collaboratives across the country are already moving in this direction. My hope is that this protocol provides some support to their efforts and makes it easier for others who are just getting started.

The HPP acknowledges the fundamental health needs first and then progresses to more clinically oriented and technologically sophisticated medical interventions. What follows is a brief description of each step of the hierarchy. All six levels of care are required for us to achieve health at the individual and collective level. Consider this version 1.0 of the protocol. I would invite you and your organization to iterate upon and advance this 1.0 version.

Healthcare Prioritization Protocol

SOCIETAL INFRASTRUCTURE

Societal infrastructure includes the most basic health needs—shelter; clothing; healthful food; safe air, water, and soil; safe, stable neighborhoods and communities; convenient access to affordable transportation; and the ability to gather socially. Within this domain, the most impactful elements in terms of healthcare utilization and costs are education, employment, and income. People with less education, employment, and income suffer ill-health and utilize high-cost healthcare resources more often. Given the evidence, it would seem that, long-term, this level of care is by far the most impactful and cost-effective.

Well-being

Well-being could be considered an "interpersonal infrastructure," as it encompasses one's emotional, relational, and social life. It describes how one is connected to one's own purpose and meaning as well as how one is connected to others in the community. This rung is about vitality and energy. It's about how much control, mastery, and autonomy one has; how much resilience one has to face life's challenges. Unfortunately, well-being along with social infrastructure is largely, if not completely, overlooked in healthcare today. Social isolation and loneliness also fall into this category as one of the most insidious and devastating epidemics of our time.

Wellness

Wellness, as I've defined it, refers specifically to physical well-being: nutrition, physical activity and movement, sleep hygiene, and the avoidance of toxins like cigarette smoking, tobacco, excess alcohol, and opiates.

Clinical Primary Prevention

Primary prevention includes screenings for cancer—mammograms for breast cancer, colonoscopies for colon cancer, Pap smears for cervical cancer. It also includes genetic screenings for predispositions to hereditary diseases and genetically driven reactions to pharmacologics. A major element in primary prevention is dental care, which, without question, is not only pertinent to dental hygiene and health, but also has an impact on one overall's health and wellness. This level of care also includes preventive immunizations.

Chronic-Disease Management

The next priority on the HPP is secondary prevention or chronic-disease management. Disease management is about maintaining health as optimally as possible despite existing medical conditions. Some examples of chronic conditions that would fall into this category are high blood pressure, diabetes, depression and anxiety, epilepsy, congestive heart failure, emphysema, asthma, and rheumatoid arthritis. Some conditions, such as Parkinson's and dementia are considered degenerative, in that they worsen over time. Others are acute in onset, such as stroke and heart attack. As medical science and treatment advances, we will learn how to overcome the degenerative nature of many of these conditions and some will likely become reversible. Chronic disease now represents the vast majority of healthcare encounters, far surpassing infection or trauma, both in the US and globally; and the costs are staggering. This rung of the HPP likely represents the greatest immediate and most proximal opportunity for improving health and reducing avoidable costs.

Acute Care

Finally, the last level of the HPP is acute and/or intensive intervention. This category includes high-tech surgical interventions, radiologic interventions, and intensive and costly chemo-therapeutics. This category also includes surgical interventions for degenerative joint diseases like knee, hip, shoulder, and back surgery, and high-tech treatment for premature births. It is clearly the costliest, the most resource-intensive, and the riskiest of healthcare domains. It is also another domain that has great opportunity for cost avoidance through the prevention of inappropriate overutilization as well as greater optimization and standardization of pre-, intra- and post-interventional protocols of care (i.e., bundles of care).

GUIDELINES ON HOW TO USE THE HPP

There are a few key points to keep in mind when deploying the HPP. I propose using the HPP as a guide, a prioritized checklist for conducting regularly scheduled environmental scans within your organization, your community, and across whatever domain of healthcare you have influence.

1. Notice that the upper three priorities on the HPP are clearly recognizable as clinical in nature. The bottom three are much less so. It's important to keep in mind the close relationship between the top half and bottom half, in that a major effort on the lower three reduces the need for the top three.

2. Up until very recently, healthcare has been defined in a way that does not typically recognize, resource, or organize the bottom three domains. If we are interested in optimal health outcomes and optimized use of resources, we must concern ourselves with the non-traditional healthcare domains. The point of this hierarchy is that appropriate healthcare should *start* at the bottom and work its way up.

3. If we're going to create an effective, efficient, and sustainable healthcare system—one that begins at the base of this hierarchy—we're going to have to start by resourcing these basic SDOH domains. This will require that we include other stakeholders in our traditional approach to healthcare. If housing is seen as a healthcare issue, then we'll need professionals working in healthcare who are housing experts. If education and employment are similarly viewed, then we're going to need professionals in healthcare who have those areas of expertise. There is a huge opportunity

for professionals with expertise in wellness, well-being, and social infrastructure. What's exciting is that we can imagine and develop healthcare collaborations that didn't exist before, including unprecedented collaborations between corporate entities, municipalities, social services, and traditional healthcare stakeholders.

Funding and resourcing social services is a political issue. Instead of avoiding that reality, let's address it head on. Attending to the bottom three foundational steps of the HPP will allow us to mitigate the current crippling cost of healthcare for individuals, families, municipalities, employers, and corporations. The bottom three foundational elements of the HPP are economic stabilizers. Our healthcare costs currently place corporate America at a competitive disadvantage on the global market. Resourcing these is an economic necessity in which corporate America wins, our federal and state governments win, our municipalities win, and our emerging and future generations win. Far from being disruptive to our commerce, attending to these three foundational elements of healthcare create whole new sectors within the healthcare industry, leading to numerous opportunities for meaningful and value-laden employment.

4. The investment of time is greatest at the bottom of the HPP. It only requires a few hours to perform a surgical procedure or a few weeks to months to treat someone with chemotherapy. But it may take years of foresight and investment to make an impact on societal, wellness, and well-being influencers. Infrastructures take time to build. The time to get a return-on-investment may be one of

the reasons why we've avoided addressing these health-care domains. But, the time frame for seeing the positive impact of healthcare in these longer-range domains also extends farther into the future. These healthcare services will pay dividends for decades to come through providing our younger generations with education, employment, and well-being. They require a commitment not just to the immediate moment, but to the future—our own, as well as that of future generations. These fundamental healthcare services also require a value-based leadership commitment to communities.

5.   The movement up the HPP represents a cost escala-tion. The preventive interventions at the bottom are less intensive clinically, medically, technologically, and for the most part, financially. As we neglect the bottom domains, we escalate the need for the domains at the top of the HPP. It's easy to ignore the foundational elements, but doing so has led to the reliance on higher-cost interventions. Due to how payment and compensation work in our health-care system, there is a profound financial incentive for the medical/industrial complex to move up the hierarchy to the high-tech, highly intensive clinical domains. From a purely humanistic or personal perspective, most would prefer treatment that fits squarely into the bottom three steps. It's far less invasive, far less risky, and far less costly.

If we're going to create something truly new and positively disruptive, we collectively need to be working on every one of these domains, and we need to reprioritize a significant amount of effort and resources to the bottom three. This reframed healthcare hierarchy allows us to take a proactive approach because it reminds us that creating a sustainable and holistic healthcare system has its roots in addressing basic human psycho-social needs. The current imbalance is clear.

With all payers shifting from fee-for-service to value-based, population-based payment, healthcare organizations will be required to make solving the SDOH a basic requirement and core set of capabilities. There are numerous healthcare systems that are understanding this need to advance the SDOH, and collaborations and coalitions forming to address it as well. What follows is one example of many that illustrates what this reframed healthcare approach might look like. What's encouraging is that the SDOH reframe movement is also being advanced by insurers, employers, and government. It's highly likely that what will be required are multi-stakeholder collaborations that include providers, payers, employers, and the government.

SDOH Reframe in Action— Geisinger Health

Geisinger Health is a bold example of an SDOH reframe that highlights how an organization that follows the steps of the Reframe Roadmap and Marketing Mindset can be successful in creating a new and better healthcare system. Like other visionary systems across the country, they've set sail on a whole new reframe adventure in healthcare delivery. They are turning the concept of the hospital inside out.

The fundamental shift driving Geisinger's strategy is the SDOH reframe. Now, Geisinger is not ignoring all the initiatives that the other leading healthcare systems are working on, such as quality and safety, appropriate utilization, clinical protocols, consumer experience, digital health, genomics, and personalized health. But what

Geisinger is doing is attacking these challenges using the powerful SDOH lever. Geisinger has been focusing its primary organizational efforts and resources on improving nutrition, physical activity, housing, transportation, and social isolation and loneliness while reducing unhealthful behaviors such as smoking, excessive alcohol consumption, and substance dependence/abuse. They are also focused on integrating mental health and genomic testing into primary preventive care.

It's simple, straightforward and common sensical, but, it's also hugely courageous. The folks at Geisinger set out to completely disrupt themselves. They are becoming a "health" company. Their stated goal is to eliminate the need for the hospital, to keep people healthy at home and in their communities rather than to focus on maximizing "heads in beds"—an industry term used to describe hospital inpatient volume. Their goal is to reduce the footprint of the hospital as it stands today and redeploy as many of their professionals and staff to different types of work that align with their key reframes of consumer-oriented, value-based care and the SDOH. Geisinger has an advantage in the value-based realm, because it is also a health plan—a payvider—the benefits of which we discussed in chapter 9. I suspect, given their legacy of true leadership, that they would pursue this path even if they weren't a payvider. And, the reality is that our current payment models are rapidly moving in the direction of risk-based, value-based payment anyway. Geisinger, to borrow hockey hall-of-famer Wayne Gretzke's well-worn phrase, is "skating quickly toward where the puck is going."

Below are descriptions of some of Geisinger's major initiatives, all derivatives of the SDOH reframe.

FRESH FOOD FARMACY

It's widely accepted that many diseases are a function of poor nutrition and dietary habits. A shocking statistic shared by Dr. David Feinberg (Geisinger's current outgoing CEO) is that when he was born in 1962, the chances of him developing type 2 diabetes in the US were 1 out of 100. For a child born in the US today, in 2019, the chances of getting type 2 diabetes are 1 in 3.[106] When I was training to be an internal-medicine physician in the late 1980s, type 2 diabetes was relatively uncommon. Today, it affects over 10 percent of the US population. Keep in mind that our genetic makeup has not changed in the past forty or fifty years. But our nutrition and our physical activity has, which is the reason we're witnessing a national epidemic of this and other chronic metabolic diseases.

From a cost perspective, the numbers are alarming. On average, a person with diabetes will have a total medical cost over twice that of someone without it. And if there are any complications from diabetes, costs can climb up to three or four times that of an individual without it. An individual with diabetes averages approximately $14,000 per year.[107] An individual with any complication from diabetes can cost well over $20,000 per year,[108] and those with severe diabetic complications can cost ten times that amount per year.[109] The typical approach to diabetes has involved treatment with medications—pills and insulin, usually prescribed by a primary-care doctor and/or a diabetologist/endocrinologist. There is some focus on diet and physical activity, and diabetologists sometimes have nutritionists working with them, or refer to nutritionists. But these nutritionists typically are office-based and can only provide basic teaching and handouts. What keeps that from being effective is that a significant percentage of the population doesn't know how to shop for or prepare healthy foods, can't afford them, or doesn't live anywhere near places to get them.

Realizing this, using its electronic health-record database, Geisinger screened all their healthcare customers who have diabetes for "food insecurity"—the inability to afford or access healthy foods. They offer these folks a "fresh food farmacy" program where they can pick up a weekly supply of fresh fruits, vegetables, and lean meats— free of charge. They also offer free classes on how to shop for healthy foods and how to prepare them for themselves and their families.[110] [111]And it's working. Even within three or four months—according to both Dr. Feinberg and Dominic Moffa, Geisinger's chief strategy officer—they've seen abnormally high blood sugars drop and HbA1c levels go from over 10 percent down to 7 percent (normal non-diabetes HbA1c levels are below 7).[112] They've also seen huge cost savings, with annual medical costs for folks with diabetes dropping from $200,000 to $40,000.[113] By some time in 2019, they expect to have served over 1.5 million meals.[114]

TRANSPORTATION

One of the most significant social determinants of health is social isolation and loneliness, and the related issue of lack of accessible and affordable transportation. If you can't easily get to friends, family, community centers, or your place of worship, it's far more likely you will struggle with feelings of isolation and loneliness. There's a substantial body of literature that demonstrates the highly negative impact of loneliness on health. Our previous US surgeon general, Dr. Vivek Murthy, likens "loneliness" to the most significant chronic disease and co-morbidity factor of our times.[115] It not only leads to greater depression and use of pain medications and alcohol but is also a major factor in making other chronic diseases worse. In fact, the literature suggests that social isolation is more harmful and costlier than diabetes or obesity, and has the comparable negative impact of smoking fifteen cigarettes a day.[116]

Realizing the implications of loneliness on health, Geisinger now offers free transportation to its customers—no questions asked. That's transportation anywhere: to the supermarket or to church, to visit grandchildren, to a local community center, or to the doctor. Geisinger's guiding belief is that if they can reduce social isolation and loneliness by providing transportation and connecting people, they're going to see not only happier people with more fulfilled and meaningful lives, but also tremendous savings in terms of improved health and lower overall medical costs. The social-isolation initiative clearly dovetails with and supports their fresh-foods efforts, because often people don't have the means to get to a food store with fresh fruits and vegetables. It also supports their initiatives to reduce alcoholism and opioid dependence and to improve mental health. If people are lonely and isolated—if they lack meaning and purpose in their lives—it's far more likely for them to resort to alcohol and recede into other substance dependence and far more likely for them to rebound into depression.

SUBSTANCE DEPENDENCE, THE OPIOID CRISIS, AND MENTAL HEALTH

Opioid dependence is a national crisis. Approximately fifty thousand people a year die from opioid overdose in the US. It's an epidemic, generated in large part by the US healthcare system itself and an ugly underside of the pharmaceutical and medical industrial complex. The 2018 statistics from the Centers for Disease Control reveal that death rates have increased significantly for Americans in the following age ranges: an increase of 8 percent for fifteen to twenty-four year-olds;

11 percent for twenty-five to thirty-four year-olds; and 7 percent for thirty-five to forty-four year-olds.[117] The victims of substance abuse are young, in the prime of their life,[118] and in the prime of their opportunity to contribute to society. Another related statistic to this crisis: the suicide rate in the US has risen by over 30 percent in half of the country and climbed to over forty-seven thousand this past year, an increase of over 3 percent.[119] That translates to approximately one American committing suicide every twelve minutes. These mortality and suicide statistics are linked to substance abuse, but the research literature has labelled this "a crisis of despair," underscoring the need for attention to the social determinants of health and the need for a reprioritization of our approach to healthcare.[120]

Geisinger's multi-pronged approach to this crisis includes a behavioral medication-assisted therapy (MAT) program that provides both therapy and medication to assist people in getting off, and staying off, of opiates. They also have a surgical "prehab" program to reduce the need for pain meds after surgery. The program seeks to rapidly improve people's health status prior to surgery, to minimize their recovery time and the need for opiates post-operatively.

Recognizing that mental health is an integral part of primary care and that the prevalence of depression, anxiety, and other behavioral issues is high, Geisinger has embedded a mental-health professional into each of their primary-care practices. Instead of the prior inconvenient and lengthy referral process, the primary-care provider can do a warm, same-day hand-off to a behavioral health colleague in the office. And following the "proven-care" approach, for which Geisinger is famous, its behavioral-health specialists are trained to follow optimized protocols. When Geisinger's leadership talks about enhancing the hope of individuals in the community as a way to improve health and a way to combat opioid dependence and alcohol-ism, they are referencing these concrete, straightforward approaches.

SPRINGBOARD HEALTHY SCRANTON INITIATIVE

Geisinger has selected a town of seventy-five thousand citizens: Scranton, Pennsylvania.[121] It's a typical town in the sense that it's come upon some economic hard times and has all of the associ-ated social problems—from poverty to violence, to drug abuse, and overall relatively poor population health. Geisinger's intention is to frame up, redesign, and organize a reproducible model of community healthcare in Scranton that can be deployed in other communi-ties around the country and around the globe. To accomplish this, the company has assembled a task force of internal healthcare and SDOH experts combined with local community leaders, education leaders, social-service-agency leaders, and successful entrepreneurs. It's a great example of the "hospital-turned-inside-out" as well as a multi-stakeholder collaboration. Their focus is not on "fixing" healthcare but on reframing it. In addition, they're applying all their population-based analytics to identify patients and families with care gaps and markers of disease.

We've spent a fair amount of time on the Geisinger story, but that's not because it's the only one of its kind. Fortunately, there are dozens, if not hundreds of examples of provider groups, payers and employers implementing SDOH-based initiatives. But, the Geisinger example does demonstrate the power of reframing from a consumer-centric Marketing Mindset, and the profound, positive impact of prioritizing SDOH as a major reframe in healthcare delivery.

The Need for Leadership

> *The social determinants of health reframe is one of the most positive, disruptive interventions we can make in our time.*

I believe the SDOH reframe is one of the most positive, disruptive interventions we can make in our time. It will require new expertise and a clear redirection of resources. It will also require that leadership and management follow the steps of the Reframe Roadmap and Marketing Mindset. Anything less than that will result in delayed substantive action and suboptimal outcomes.

The most essential component, however, goes beyond roadmaps and resources to the determination of a new type of leadership: a coalition of value-based leadership. Up until now, we typically think of leaders as individuals, often with supportive teams and focused on responsibility for a singular entity, organization, or corporation. The leadership required for the SDOH reframe is one that will assume responsibility for a more broadly impactful set of goals. The next generation of leaders will be called to focus not just on the successful outcomes of their own organizations but on the successful outcomes of their community and country.

> *The leadership required for the social determinants of health reframe is one that will assume responsibility for a more broadly impactful set of goals.*

We are, I believe, witnessing the emergence of this type of leadership—courageous, strategic, disruptive leaders who have a broader vision of what is needed to transform healthcare. Most of the people I've referred to in this book demonstrate this type of leadership in their *reorienting, redefining,* and *redirecting* of health-care into one that is more value-based, customer-oriented, and community-focused.

One example of this sort of leadership—along the lines of the SDOH reframe—is the Healthcare Anchor Network, a national collaborative of healthcare systems sharing best practices for iden-tifying and addressing SDOH and sharing a policy and commu-nications platform to effect change across the nation. The Health Anchor Network was created through the partnership of Robert Wood Johnson Saint Barnabas—the largest healthcare system in New Jersey, Kaiser Permanente, and Pro Medica.[122] The Network has now grown to over forty health systems including, not surprisingly, Geisinger. Its goal is to document and codify the combined efforts of the participants so that these can be scaled and spread to others both nationally and internationally.[123]

Conclusion

We have a long way to go when it comes to understanding, identify-ing, addressing, and solving for the SDOH. Even as I write these words, I'm reminded of a comment Michellene Davis (EVP and chief corporate affairs officer at Robert Wood Johnson Saint Barnabas) made during one of our discussions: "Knowing what we know, shouldn't we be eliminating these health inequities and disparities, not just reducing them?" The examples in this section offer encourag-ing evidence that the SDOH reframe finally has legs; but clearly there is much that still needs to be done. Overwhelmingly, our current focus still resides predominantly on the clinically-oriented aspects of healthcare. In many ways, it's understandable. But, if it's already so widely understood and accepted that the vast majority of the opportunity and impact we could have on health are a function of SDOH, why aren't we spending more time and effort on those factors? Why aren't we diverting more of our resources to them? And why aren't we forming more hard-hitting, goal-oriented networks and coalitions, not just to address these challenges, but to resolve them? These are questions for and of leadership. They are the questions that this pivotal, historic moment in healthcare is asking of our leaders. These are questions that call for action and for a reframing of leadership.

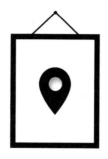

A CALL TO ACTION

*Commitment is the intentional choice to eliminate all other choices
except for the choice to move forward. A leader intentionally
creates the environment where only one choice is possible...*

—**Cort Dial,** *Heretics to Heroes, A Memoir on Modern Leadership*

The purpose of this book is to provide leaders with a reliable and replicable roadmap for creating positive, disruptive change in healthcare. A roadmap implies that there is a desired destination and outcome. It implies something about making the journey easier, more directed, and more purposeful. Roadmaps increase the likelihood of getting there and reduce the time it takes to get there. This book is written to

> *The purpose of this book is to provide leaders with a reliable and replicable roadmap for creating positive, disruptive change in healthcare.*

assist leaders who are interested in getting there in the most efficient way possible. It's written for leaders who are interested in changing the game; leaders who are dedicated to transforming healthcare.

The Reframe Roadmap and Marketing Mindset comprise the major steps required for healthcare transformation. If we intend to transition into a sustainable, value-based industry, we will need to *reorient* our thinking, *redefine* our problems, and *redirect* our strategies, tactics, and resources. If we intend to create consumer-centric organizations, products, and services, we will need to *rebrand* from within an empathetic, demand-side perspective with focused and explicit value propositions; *redesign* for an extremely engaging and relevant experience as well as for *results* that really matter to consumers; and *reorganize* for synergies that emancipate the tremendous value potential currently locked up in our constraining constructs. We cannot ignore or skip any of these steps if our goal is to have a thriving system of healthcare, and for us to thrive within as a result of that system. There are no shortcuts, quick fixes, or technologic "shiny-object" solutions that will accomplish our stated goals. Without the combined steps of the Reframe Roadmap and the Marketing Mindset, the journey will continue to be frustrating, the destination prolonged, and the appropriate life-saving and life-enhancing outcomes suboptimal.

The key component to a successful journey, however, is *leadership*—a brand of leadership that believes it's better to disrupt oneself than to be disrupted by others. I believe that if audacious leaders and leadership teams adopt the Reframe Roadmap and Marketing Mindset as well as the SDOH reframe, we could transform healthcare at a much-accelerated pace, and on a much larger scale. I also believe that the approach outlined in this book offers a profound competitive advantage to those who deploy it. We've spent the past few decades witnessing new trends and tactics that mostly attempt to reengineer healthcare, which has led to proximal improvement. Reframing, on the other hand, is an approach that leads to transformative change.

There is little doubt that healthcare is rapidly moving in the direction of consumerism—what might even be considered a consumer healthcare revolution. One of the greatest benefits of the Reframe Roadmap and the Marketing Mindset is that they offer leaders, managers, and practitioners in healthcare the means to shift our deeply held beliefs about patients and payers—and advance an approach on how to become customer-centric. Along these lines, the reframes that I've introduced in this book reflect the type of healthcare that each and every one of us would want for ourselves, our families, our friends, and our communities. At the core of all our efforts to reframe healthcare are the goals of quality, safety, reliability, consistency, convenience, access, compassion, service, and affordability; delivering the specific outcomes that matter to consumers, and—so importantly—affording people the respect and dignity they deserve.

Most everyone in healthcare today is attempting to do the right thing in a system fraught with cultural and financial challenges and tensions. The context of our administrative leadership, as well as our general legacy healthcare culture, is one of conservatism and tight integration. Administrative and clinical leaders, practicing clinicians, and support staff must all be focused and do their best to keep the trains running on time and on the right track. This is no minor feat. There is always critically complex and highly technical clinical work being performed, and there is little room for error. There are no holidays or time-outs in healthcare and few opportunities for do-overs.

At the periphery of this tightly managed and regulated system, there is a burgeoning counterculture—one of innovation, entrepreneurship, and disruption. There are individuals, teams, and organizations that want to solve bigger problems and achieve unprecedented value for their customers. At this moment, we need both cultures to be superbly functional and collaborative, even if they are on different paths. The Reframe Roadmap is an approach that acknowledges both cultures. It bridges these divergent paths by serving as a template for helping leaders hold the tension between what's needed for immediate safety, effectiveness, and efficiency; and what's necessary for continuous iteration, rapid disruptive change, and large-scale deployment.

This may be derived from an evolutionary survival instinct—our ingrained belief that inaction or delayed action is inherently safer than action. While this may be true under relatively stable circumstances, in times of rapid change and upheaval, our evolutionary wiring becomes a liability. Inaction may be a maneuver for surviving but it is certainly not an approach for thriving. As Adam Grant writes in his book, *Originals: How Non-Conformists Move the World*, "...in the long run, research shows that the mistakes we regret are not errors of commission, but errors of omission. If we could do things over, most of us would censor ourselves less and express our ideas more." Coming at it from the perspective of social justice, Martin Luther King Jr. said, in a sermon on courage, "A man dies when he refuses to stand up for that which is right. A man dies when he refuses to stand up for justice. A man dies when he refuses to take a stand for that which is true."

In applying these teachings to the state of healthcare delivery today, it is my hope that this book has provided you with: (1) A sense of urgency and an understanding of the need to reframe and reorient our thinking; (2) a template from which to interpret the foundational causal forces driving the game-changing trends in the market, including the social determinants of health reframe; (3) an appreciation of the powerful role that employers and corporate America will play in catalyzing and participating in the transformation of healthcare; (4) an understanding of the value-laden market shift that is already well underway toward segmented and hyper-segmented healthcare brands, linked by coordinating platforms; (5) a supportive guide (and the steps required) for generating and translating new ideas into sustainable and scalable customer-oriented products and services.

> *The ultimate purpose of the Reframe Roadmap and Marketing Mindset is to humanize healthcare.*

There are numerous "revolutions" afoot in healthcare today. But successful revolutions require solid principles, visionary leadership, and a well-aligned plan. This roadmap provides us with the principles and the plan. The leadership and deployment are up to you.

As I mentioned in the Introduction to this book, the ultimate purpose of the Reframe Roadmap and Marketing Mindset is to humanize healthcare. To humanize it for those who serve within the system, and of course, for those who are served by the system. Few generations are given the opportunity to create significant progressive change in an area as vital as national and

> *This moment in healthcare history is calling for pioneering leaders to change the trajectory of healthcare in the US.*

global health. Few generations are given the opportunity to rectify long-standing health inequities and disparities, and to profoundly impact and advance the health and welfare of generations to come. We have been given these opportunities.

There are several weighty responsibilities on the shoulders of healthcare leaders, particularly at this point in time. One of them is restoring the trust of our customers and our providers. The role of leadership today is not just to provide healthcare, but to restore trust in our integrity, authenticity, and motivation; in our honesty and transparency; and in our competence. What this moment in healthcare history is calling for—what our customers, communities, corporations, and country are calling for—are pioneering leaders who are called to and compelled to change the trajectory of healthcare in the US.

Consider this book an invitation to embark upon the Reframe Roadmap—an invitation to be an active participant in this historic moment in healthcare. But, like most invitations, the time to reply will come and go. How are you going to respond?

I've mentioned this quote once before in the course of this book, and I'll repeat it here, again, to drive home this call-to-action. Peter Drucker—one of the founders and most eclectic thought leaders of modern management—wrote, "The greatest danger in times of turbulence is not the turbulence; it is to act with yesterday's logic." This is a great time to be in healthcare for those excited by the purpose and the potential of generating a new logic to steer us out of these turbulent times.

Consider this book an invitation to embark upon the Reframe Roadmap—an invitation to be an active participant in this historic moment in healthcare. But, like most invitations, the time to reply will come and go. How are you going to respond?

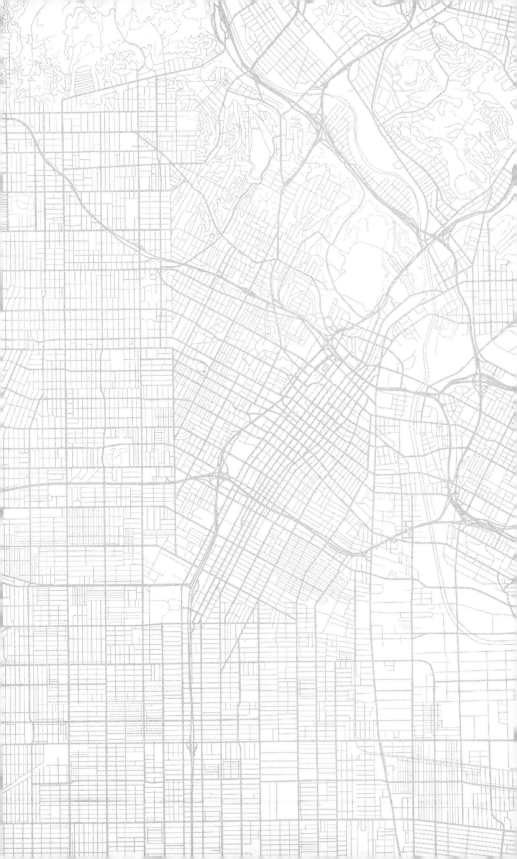

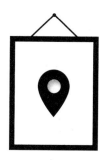

ACKNOWLEDGMENTS

First, I would like to thank my wife, Dr. Lisa Davidson, who in addition to being one of the best physicians I have ever met, is also a loving partner and mother. Lisa has given me tremendous latitude over the past two or three years, allowing me to spend thousands of hours—evenings, weekends and on vacations—working on this book as well as on the podcast series. I also must thank her for the profound wisdom and guidance she has provided me at critical times along this journey. I respect, trust and value her opinion tremendously. Her knowledge, intelligence, and wisdom are beyond anything I will ever achieve, and her kindness, generosity and good humor is a gift not only to us, her family, but also to her friends, colleagues and community. There is no way I could have pursued or completed this book without her patience and support. There is no way I can express my appreciation and love for her.

Second, I need to mention and thank my children, Emily and Jacob. They are, as I've told them from the moment they could understand, the only gift in life I ever really wanted. Over the past couple of years, I have often thought about the Harry Chapin song, "Cats in the Cradle," as I spent much too much time focused on the book instead of on my son and daughter. It is without question, the greatest sacrifice I've made in this endeavor. There were numerous times over the past couple of years when I wanted to go for a walk, or throw a ball, or go on a bike ride, or just play ping pong with the kids, but instead, I forced myself to sit in the chair at the desk in my study and write. I want to thank Emily and Jacob for their understanding and apologize for the many times I was distracted by this book, and the podcast. I will try to figure out how to be better at this. One solace (perhaps rationale) I have on this account is that they have witnessed first-hand this example of pursuing and completing a project as serious, complex, and overwhelming as the writing and publishing of a book as well as the lesson of what it means to be committed to a higher purpose and pursuit.

Third, without question, the most gratifying part of the book writing experience has been the awesome individuals who this project has given me access to. The podcasting and the book writing have provided me with an excuse and introduction to speak to and correspond with stellar human beings, and to consider them as colleagues and friends.

Picking up on this issue of colleagues and friends, I'd like to thank all of the *leaders* and *heroes* that I've interviewed for the podcast. These interviews, and the relationships that have emerged, have been the most rewarding experience of my entire career—perhaps, with the one exception of directly providing medical care to patients and their families. These podcast dialogues, as well as numerous non-recorded dialogues, served as the qualitative research for this book. But to characterize these interviews as only "research" falls far short of the experience. Someone recently asked me how I selected the people I've interviewed, who ended up getting posted online. I responded without hesitation, "I fall in love with them—with who they are and what they're doing. I fall in love with their purpose, their passion, their persistence and above all else, their commitment to making the world so much better than it is." It's fair to say that I adore these individuals who have been featured on the podcast:

Tom Charland, Cathryn Gunther, Bob Matthews, Hesky Kutscher, Joanna Strober, Par Bolina MD, Devin Gross, Rushika Fernandoulle MD, Eyal Gura, Don Berwick MD, Sean Duffy, John Moore MD, Stuart Levine MD, Sara Vaezy, Aaron Martin, Robert Andrews, Sami Inkinen, Mike McSherry, Len D'Avolio PhD, Kyra Bobinet MD, Alex Coren, Christina Dempsey, Richard Baron MD, Dave Chase, Glenn Steele MD, Barbara McAneny MD, Raphaela O'Day PhD, Josh Luke PhD, Dave Slawson MD, Scott Becker, Dominic Moffa, Al Lewis, Mark Briesacher MD, Kevin Volpp MD, Chris Chen MD, Michellene Davis Esq, Samir Damani MD, Andy Edeburn, Shreya Kangovi MD, Zack Cooper PhD, Kevan Mabbutt, Robert Pearl MD, Harold Paz MD, Marcus Osborne, David Contorno, and Jeff Thompson MD. There are others at the time of this writing whom I've interviewed or am about to interview for the podcast, and just haven't had a chance to post yet. These remarkable individuals include: Patrick Conway MD, Jay Desai, Karen Horgan, Sachin Jain MD, David Michael Levine MD, Valerie Monet, Bob Moesta, Mitesh Patel MD, Rita Numerof PhD, Glen Tullman, Karen Horgan, and Scott Weingarten MD.

I'd also like to thank mentors who have been beyond generous with their time and wisdom—too many to mention, but a few stand out for me, especially in the writing of this book. The first person is someone I've admired for decades: Dr. Don Berwick. Don is one of the most courageous, brilliant, humanistic, and accomplished healthcare leaders of our time. Despite his well-deserved international recognition and the incredible demands on his time and attention, he has always been incredibly responsive and giving to me. I just can't thank him enough for what he means to me, his amazing body of work, and his contribution to healthcare and humanity.

I've never met anyone quite like Scott Becker. He is so accomplished, productive, and generative—yet so humble and generous with his time and his wisdom. Despite how much he's got on his plate, whenever I've called or emailed Scott for advice, he'll get back within a few hours, or a couple of days at most. And more than that, whenever we've spoken, he's never been rushed or distracted.

Every once in a while, you come across an individual who influences your life in ways you couldn't ever predict. Bob Moesta is one of those people for me. Bob is a student and disciple of professor Clayton Christensen of the Harvard Business School. He's also a scholar, engineer, and management consultant of extraordinary talent and skill. I had the privilege of working with him on a project three or so years ago. The experience was inspiring and catalytic. Working with Bob helped me find my own voice.

The most recent mentor I've had the incredibly good fortune of meeting is Stephen Martin, introduced to me by my good friend, Cathryn Gunther. Steve is the former CEO of BCBS of Nebraska. He's one of the most brilliant and experienced minds I've come across in healthcare. His comprehension and assimilation of the complexities of healthcare delivery is astounding. I can listen to him for hours.

There are other mentors I could spend paragraphs describing; but, for now, I want to take a moment to recognize and sincerely thank a few people who have inspired, supported and educated me along the way. Their example has guided my thinking and actions. A huge debt of gratitude to these courageous leaders and generous teachers: Tom Bodenheimer MD, Robert Fritz, Carl Isihara MD, Gene Lindsey MD, Ed Noffsinger PhD, and Tony Suchman MD.

I'd like to also thank all of the professors and instructors that are part of the "Masters in Healthcare Management" Physician Executive Program at the Harvard T.H. Chan School of Public Health. That two-year experience was a turning point in my career. It wasn't just the instructors, but also my fellow students, who were all so highly experienced and accomplished. There are too many names to mention but I am compelled to thank professor Nancy M. Kane, who is one of the most brilliant strategic thinkers I've ever met, and whose talent in teaching case studies has always astounded me. I must also thank Linda MacCracken, who taught the marketing course from which the thesis for the book was born; and Rick Siegrist who not only taught us cost accounting and entrepreneurship, but also taught us how to have fun in our work.

I want to sincerely thank my amazing friends and colleagues, who over the past couple of years have thrown me a lifeline when I've needed it most. I apologize ahead of time if I've inadvertently left someone out here: Amy Barry, Justin Batt, Par Bolina, Jim Boswell, Tony Burke, Michael Cantor, Alisahah Cole, Tom Charland, Len D'Avolio, Genevieve Fairbrother, Lisa Gianferante, Cathryn Gunther, Sachin Gupta, Priti Lakhani, Tom Laymon, David Levine, John Lewis, Josh Luke, Steve Martin, Bob Matthews, George McLendon, Dan Murrey, Brad Power, Scott Rissmiller, Jim Rivenbark MD, Mike Ruhlen, Geoffrey Rose, John Santopietro, Leo Spector, Harold Sturner, Bob Tavares, Tim Simard, Josh Vire, and Greg Weidner. I want each one to know that I think of them often and can't thank them enough for their friendship, their generosity, and for the example they provide me. And a note of gratitude to Tom Charland, Alisahah Cole, Cathryn Gunther, Linda MacCracken, Steve Martin, Dan Murrey, Scott Rissmiller, Geoffrey Rose, and Greg Weidner for reviewing sections of the manuscript along the way.

I want to thank my sister, Estee Neuwirth. Estee is a sociologist by training with post-doctoral credentials and has been applying her world-class skills at Kaiser Permanente for nearly thirteen years. We have developed a relationship as true colleagues—comparing notes on our work in redesigning healthcare. I've learned so much from Estee over the past decade—about ethnography, human centered design thinking and care redesign in general—and can't thank her enough. I also want to thank my brother, Michael, who is a superbly gifted and innovative interventional radiologist. He's always been an advocate for being agile and courageous with one's life and career, urging me not to waste my time or effort in places it's not appreciated. Almost every major move I've made in my life has required a motivating heart-to-heart talk with my brother Michael. My youngest sister, Jacqueline, is a soulful artist. I've learned so many lessons from her about creativity and expression, and continue to draw inspiration from her evolving mastery in photography and painting. Her talent and her portfolio are remarkable, and provided me with an example in creating this book. My father, Arieh (Leo) Neuwirth, is a force to be reckoned with. He recently retired from his career as a mechanical and electrical engineer—having worked fifty-eight years in one job—and being exceptionally (and I mean *exceptionally*) productive until literally the day he retired. My Dad, from the moment I can remember, has taught us to treat every human being with deep respect and dignity—to remember that every person is someone's son or daughter. I can distinctly remember when I was a child, sitting for minutes in the car (somewhat exasperated) while my Dad would chat with the attendants at the gas station. He always made the time to chitchat (kibbitz) with anyone and everyone, whether to provide advice or just lend an empathetic ear. I had the phrase, "everyone puts their pants on one leg at a time" emblazoned in my psyche as a young child. It's a lesson I will never forget, and one I carried with me into the hospital wards as a resident, and into my medical practice, as well as into my management and executive roles. Dad sees something positive in everyone, and I suspect I gained my deep-rooted sense of appreciation for other people's potential from him. My Dad also constantly demonstrated to us the healing power of humor. I'm fortunate to have been raised by two parents who created a loving, caring, and safe home. I don't take that for granted.

I want to thank all of the podcast listeners—especially those that take the time to email and provide feedback and suggestions. I can't tell you how seriously I take your feedback and appreciate you taking the time out of your busy days to write and chat with me. I'd also like to mention and thank James Harden, who has been my sound engineer since I first began recording the podcasts. His skill and experience has saved me on numerous occasions. His guidance and wisdom continue to influence my thinking. I'd also like to thank Caroline Arey, who has worked with me from the beginning to post the podcasts and the emails I send out weekly. It's hard to describe what it means to be able to trust someone with something that is so important to me.

I owe an incredible debt of gratitude to Jess Greenwood. Jess is part of the 3 SMS team that I've used as exclusive social media consultants for the past year. She and her colleagues, Lisa Gualtieri and Sandra Rosenbluth, do an awesome job. As I was struggling between the third and fourth rewriting of this book, I needed an outstanding editor that understood healthcare and whose judgement I could trust implicitly. It suddenly dawned on me that perhaps Jess could help. What I didn't realize was how much editorial and writing skill she possessed, or the depth of her healthcare knowledge and judgement. I'm not sure I would have finished this book on time if Jess hadn't joined me for the final leg of journey. We worked at a relentless pace for months as I literally rewrote the book from start to finish. Jess kept pace and never let me down. I simply can't thank her enough and look forward to our continuing collaboration.

Along a similar line, I am so deeply grateful to Rich Hill, who has been my career and life coach for the past three years. Rich is an exceptional executive coach and organizational consultant. He has gotten me through some rough patches—moments of self-doubt and despair. But much more than that, he has helped me uncover so much about myself. He helped me find my voice and my direction. He taught me how to reconnect with my core truths and strip away the noise. What I admire about Rich is that he's so very real. He lives his truth, his passion, and his power in every conversation and in every interaction. I am so grateful there are people in the world like Rich whom I believe could do or be anything but decide that it's their purpose to help others become themselves. If it hadn't been for Rich, I'm not sure I would have begun speaking out again, or writing, or podcasting. I trust his skill, his judgement, and his intentions implicitly. He is a jewel, and I'm glad that he's given me the gift of his time, his attention, his heart, his mind, and his beautiful soul for these past few years.

I had another coach join for me a while: Cynthia Freeman. It was during one of the most challenging times in my career. Cynthia's bold and light spirit—and her incredibly positive attitude—was a like a light in the darkness. It was during our conversations that my idea for writing a book emerged. I feel a deep and binding gratitude to her for helping me cross that chasm. We haven't spoken in a while, but I still feel her spirit every time I think of her, and it makes me smile.

In the first few months of writing this book, I began to conduct interviews and then realized that I needed to share these interviews with others. Someone mentioned launching a podcast. I had no idea how to do that. Somehow, I tripped across a remarkable person, an MIT grad, ex-Wall Street financial wizkid named Brian Rose. He had left a high-flying career, moved to London and started to build a media empire. I had been listening to his video series, "London Real," and the interviews were entertaining and inspiring. One day, I noticed he was offering an online course on how to launch a podcast. I signed up for the course and spent my evenings and weekends during the summer of 2017 learning how to set up, launch, and maintain a podcast. It was scary—putting myself out there in that way. I had no producer, no crew, nothing—just me and an online course. Like my coach Rich Hill, Brian brings tremendous integrity to his work, and to his life. He walks his talk. I admire the independent entrepreneurial life he has carved out for himself. I don't believe I would have been able to launch the podcast if it hadn't been for Brian and his team.

I also would like to acknowledge and thank my colleagues at Atrium Health. My colleagues are wonderful individuals, and collectively, we're improving healthcare in the Carolinas and beyond. A particular shout-out to my colleagues in the Medical Group, in the Population Health division, and in the Carolinas Physician Alliance, as well as my colleagues in the Innovation Division. I learn from you all the time, and almost certainly don't thank you enough.

The effort of writing this book was a huge collective effort. I used to be an avid hiker, and although I haven't ever done serious mountain climbing, I understand that sherpas are those people who carry the load and guide the way. So, I'd like to thank the sherpa team at Advantage Media Group—Nate Best, Kristin Goodale, Kirby Anderson, Megan Elger, Jennifer Holt, Josh Houston, Patti

Boysen, Y-Danair Niehrah, Justin Batt, and all the behind-the-scenes folks. I'd also like to thank Tiarra Tompkins and Tammy Kling from OnFire Books, who gave me a much-needed boost in the last leg of the climb. Their experience and encouragement has been of incredible value to me in bringing this book to completion. I would like to call out a special "thank you" to Justin Batt. I've known Justin for years. This fellow hiker and guide on the book writing journey has a unique sense of integrity. There were many times along the climb that I would turn to him, and he always restored my sense of hope and purpose.

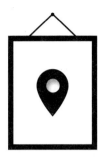

REFERENCES

Chapter 1

1   John T. James, "A New, Evidence-based Estimate of Patient Harms Associated with Hospital Care," *Journal of Patient Safety* 9, no 3 (September 2013): 122–128.

2   Marty Makary, *Unaccountable – What Hospitals Won't Tell You and How Transparency Can Revolutionize Health Care*, (Bloomsbury Press, 2012).

3   "Hospital Errors are the Third Leading Cause of Death in U.S., and New Hospital Safety Scores Show Improvements Are Too Slow," Leapfrog Hospital Safety Grade, November 18, 2018, http://www.hospitalsafetygrade.org/newsroom/display/hospitalerrors-thirdleading-causeofdeathinus-improvementstooslow.

4   Eric C. Schneider et al., "Mirror, Mirror 2017: International Comparison Reflects Flaws and Opportunities for U.S. Health Care," The Commonwealth Fund, (2017), https://interactives.commonwealthfund.org/2017/july/mirror-mirror/.

5   "Health United States, 2017 with Special Feature on Mortality," National Center for Health Statistics, 2017, https://www.cdc.gov/nchs/data/hus/hus17.pdf.

6   L. R. Woskie Papanicolas and A. K. Jha, "Health Care Spending in the United States and Other High-Income Countries," *Journal of the American Medical Association* 319, no. 10 (March 13, 2018): 1024–39.

7   Katherine E. Fleming-Dutra et al., "Prevalence of Inappropriate Antibiotic Prescriptions Among US Ambulatory Care Visits, 2010-2011," *JAMA* 315, no. 17 (2016): 1864-1873; "Antibiotic Prescribing and Use in Doctor's Offices," Centers for Disease Control and Prevention, November 7, 2018, https://www.cdc.gov/antibiotic-use/community/programs-measurement/ measuring-antibiotic-prescribing.html.

8   Holly Hedegaard, Margaret Warner, and Arialdi M. Miniño, "Drug Overdose Deaths in the United States 1999-2016," NCHS Data Brief No. 294, December 2017, https://www.cdc.gov/nchs/data/databriefs/db294.pdf.

9   "Survey: 79 Million americans Have Problems with Medical Bills or Debt," The Commonwealth Fund, https://www. commonwealthfund.org/publications/newsletter-article/ survey-79-million-americans-have-problems-medical-bills-or-debt.

10   Eric C. Schneider et al., "Health Care in America: The Experience of People with Serious Illness," http://features.commonwealthfund.org/ health-care-in-america?_ga=2.242148354.1600150041.1544900401- 312443446.1544900401The Commonwealth Fund.

11   Margot Sanger-Katz, "1,495 Americans Describe the Financial Reality of Being Really Sick," *New York Times*, October 17, 2018, https://www.nytimes. com/2018/10/17/upshot/health-insurance-severely-ill-financial-toxicity-. html.

12   Speech: Remarks by CMS Administrator Seema Verma at the HIMSS18 Conference, March 6, 2018, https://www.cms.gov/newsroom/press-releases/ speech-remarks-cms-administrator-seema-verma-himss18-conference.

13   Jeff Elton and Anne O'Riordan, *Healthcare Disrupted* (Wiley Press, 2016).

14   Ibid.

15 "Trust in Healthcare," Edelman Trust Barometer, June 2018, https://www. edelman.com/post/trust-in-healthcare-2018.

16 "Distrust in the U.S. Health System: Are We Paying Attention?" The Keckley Report, 2018, https://www.paulkeckley.com/the-keckley-report/2018/10/1/ distrust-in-the-us-health-system-are-we-paying-attention.

17 Jeffrey M. Jones and R. J. Reinhart, "Americans Remain Dissatisfied With Healthcare Costs," Gallup Well-Being, November 28, 2018, https://news. gallup.com/poll/245054/americans-remain-dissatisfied-healthcare-costs. aspx.

18 Ashley Kirzinger et al., "KFF Election Tracking Poll: Health Care in the 2018 Midterms,"Henry J. Kaiser Family Foundation, October 18, 2018, https://www.kff.org/health-reform/poll-finding/ kff-election-tracking-poll-health-care-in-the-2018-midterms.

19 :Consumerism in Healthcare with Kevin Mabbutt," Zeev Neuwirth podcast September 12, 2018, http://shoutengine.com/CreatingaNewHealthcare/ episode-45-consumerism-in-healthcare-with-kevan-ma-65683.

20 "Healthcare Professional Burnout, Depression and Suicide Prevention," American Foundation for Suicide Prevention, 2019, https://afsp.org/our-work/education/healthcare-professional-burnout-depression-suicide-prevention.

21 Eva S. Schernhammer and Graham A. Colditz, :Suicide Rates Among Physicians: A Quantitative and Gender Assessment (Meta-Analysis)," American Journal of Psychiatry 161, no. 12 (December 2004): 2295–2302.

22 "This Is Not Your Father's or Mother's AMA - the AMA's Moonshot Moment - with Barbara McAneny MD, President-elect of the American Medical Association," Zeev Neuwirth podcast, March 9, 2018, http:// shoutengine.com/CreatingaNewHealthcare/this-is-not-your-fathers-or-mothers-ama-the-ama-54287.

23   Alex M. Azar II, Remarks on Value-Based Transformation to the Federation of American Hospitals, Federation of American Hospitals, March 5, 2018; Washington, D.C., https://www.hhs.gov/about/leadership/secretary/speeches/2018-speeches/remarks-on-value-based-transformation-to-the-federation-of-american-hospitals.html.

24   "The Third Era of Medicine with Dr. Don Berwick, President Emeritus, Institute for Healthcare Improvement, Zeev Neuwirth podcast, November 5, 2017, http://shoutengine.com/CreatingaNewHealthcare/the-third-era-of-medicine-with-dr-don-berwick-pr-46122.

Chapter 2

25   Peter F. Drucker, *The Essential Drucker: The Best of Sixty Years of Peter Drucker's Essential Writings on Management,* (Harper Business, 2008).

26   Jeremy Gutsche, *Better and Faster: the Proven Path to Unstoppable Ideas,*(Crown Publishing, 2015).

27   Robert J. Lang, *Origami,* https://langorigami.com.

28   John Leach, *Survival Psychology* (MacMillan Press, 1994).

29   Arthur Koestler, *The Act of Creation* (Last Century Media, 2014).

Chapter 3

30   "Walmart's Consumer Oriented Healthcare Transformation with Marcus Osborne, Zeev Neuwirth podcast, October 25, 2018, http://shoutengine.com/CreatingaNewHealthcare/episode-48-walmarts-consumer-oriented-healthca-68068.

31   Jeremy Gutsche, *Better and Faster: the Proven Path to Unstoppable Ideas* (Crown Publishing, 2015).

32   Ron Adner, "Many Companies Still Don't Know How to Compete in the Digital Age," *Harvard Business Review*, March 28, 2016, https://hbr.org/2016/03/many-companies-still-dont-know-how-to-compete-in-the-digital-age.

Chapter 4

33   Avi Dan, "What Do You Call A 17-Year-Old Ad Campaign? Priceless," *Forbes*, August 25, 2014, https://www.forbes.com/sites/avidan/2014/08/25/what-do-you-call-a-17-year-old-ad-campaign-priceless/#f044fd17142e.

Chapter 5

34   "On-Demand Urgent Care with Tom Charland, Zeev Neuwirth podcast, August 31, 2017, http://shoutengine.com/CreatingaNewHealthcare/on-demand-urgent-care-with-tom-charland-42113.

35   Kenneth D. Kochanek et al., "Mortality in the United States, 2016," NCHS Data Brief No. 293, December 2017, https://www.cdc.gov/nchs/data/databriefs/db293.pdf

36   Ibid.

37   "Redefining & Redesigning Primary Care with Rushika Fernandopulle, CEO of Iora Health, "Zeev Neuwirth podcast, October 29, 2017, http://shoutengine.com/CreatingaNewHealthcare/redefining-redesigning-primary-care-with-rushika-45760.

38   "Affordable Concierge Primary Care - Honoring Seniors & Delivering Better Health Outcomes,"Zeev Neuwirth podcast, May 17, 2018, http://shoutengine.com/CreatingaNewHealthcare/episode-38-affordable-concierge-primary-care--5862.

39   "Digital Behavioral Medicine with Sean Duffy, Co-founder & CEO of Omada Health," Zeev Neuwirth podcast, November 7, 2017,

http://shoutengine.com/CreatingaNewHealthcare/digital-behavioral-medicine-with-sean-duffy-co-fo-46189.

40   "Digital Health with Sami Inkinen, Founder & CEO of Virta Health," Zeev Neuwirth podcast, December 3, 2017, http://shoutengine.com/CreatingaNewHealthcare/digital-health-with-sami-inkinen-founder-ceo-of-47559.

41   "Reframing chronic disease management - with George McLendon PhD, Founder of SensorRX; and VP for Therapeutics Research & Development at Atrium Health," Zeev Neuwirth podcast, February 9, 2018, http://shoutengine.com/CreatingaNewHealthcare/reframing-chronic-disease-management-with-george-51393.

42   "Digital Health with Mike McSherry, CEO of Xealth," Zeev Neuwirth podcast, December 10, 2017, http://shoutengine.com/CreatingaNewHealthcare/digital-health-with-mike-mcsherry-ceo-of-xealth-47907.

Chapter 6

43   "Walmart's consumer oriented healthcare transformation with Marcus Osborne," Zeev Neuwirth podcast, October 25, 2018, http://shoutengine.com/CreatingaNewHealthcare/episode-48-walmarts-consumer-oriented-healthca-68068.

44   Benedict Sheppard et al., "The Business Value of Design," *Mckinsey Quarterly*, (Oct 2018), https://www.mckinsey.com/~/media/McKinsey/Business%20Functions/McKinsey%20Design/Our%20insights/The%20business%20value%20of%20design/The-business-value-of-design-vF.ashx.

45   UnitedHealthcare CEO: Digital health will soon be synonymous with health Nicky Lineaweaver and Laurie Beaver, "UnitedHealthcare CEO: Digital health will soon be synonymous with health," *Business Insider*, (September 12, 2018), 2018 https://www.businessinsider.com/steve-nelson-unitedhealthcare-ceo-interview-2018-9.

46 "Infographic: Health Ambitions Study: Transforming care delivery," aetna, June 15, 2018, https://news.aetna.com/2018/06/health-ambitions-study-transforming-care-delivery.

47 Maria Castellucci, "CEO Power Panel: Health systems focus on patient-centered care as consumerism takes hold," Modern Healthcare, September 15, 2018, https://www.modernhealthcare.com/article/20180915/NEWS/180919978; Laura Lovett, "How hospitals can engage consumers to innovate a new patient experience," MobiHealthNews, September 28, 2018, https://www.mobihealthnews.com/content/how-hospitals-can-engage-consumers-innovate-new-patient-experience.

48 Stephen Klasko, "Forging a Match.com relationship with patients," *AthenaInsight*, October 23, 2017, https://www.athenahealth.com/insight/sites/insight/files/10.23%20Forging%20a%20Match.com%20relationship%20with%20patients.pdf.

49 David Wenner, "UPMC CEO: 'We desire to become the Amazon of health care'," Pennsylvania Realtime News, Nov 3, 2017, https://www.pennlive.com/news/2017/11/upmc_ceo_we_desire_to_become_t.html

50 "Consumerism in Healthcare with Kevan Mabbutt," Zeev Neuwirth podcast September 12, 2018, http://shoutengine.com/CreatingaNewHealthcare/episode-45-consumerism-in-healthcare-with-kevan-ma-65683.

51 "Consumerism in Healthcare with Kevan Mabbutt, Zeev Neuwirth podcast, September 12, 2018, http://shoutengine.com/CreatingaNewHealthcare/episode-45-consumerism-in-healthcare-with-kevan-ma-65683.

52 Mitesh S. Patel et al., "Generic Medication Prescription Rates After Health System–Wide Redesign of Default Options Within the Electronic Health Record," *Journal of the American Medical Association, Internal Medicine* 176, no. 6, (2016): 847-848, https://doi.org/10.1001/jamainternmed.2016.1691.

Chapter 7

53 "Digital Health and Behavior Change with Roy Rosin." Zeev Neuwirth podcast, December 18, 2017, http://shoutengine.com/CreatingaNewHealthcare/digital-health-and-behavior-change-with-roy-rosin-48266

54 International Consortium for Health Outcomes Measurement, ICHOM, https://www.ichom.org.

55 "Leadership Principles," Amazon Jobs, https://www.amazon.jobs/en/principles.

56 "Digital Health with Aaron Martin, Executive Vice President and Chief Digital Officer at Providence St. Joseph Health," Zeev Neuwirth podcast, November 20 2017, http://shoutengine.com/CreatingaNewHealthcare/digital-health-with-aaron-martin-executive-vice-p-46903.

57 "Consumerism in Healthcare with Kevin Mabbutt," Zeev Neuwirth podcast, September 12, 2018, http://shoutengine.com/CreatingaNewHealthcare/episode-45-consumerism-in-healthcare-with-kevan-ma-65683.

58 "The Third Era of Medicine with Dr. Don Berwick, President Emeritus, Institute for Healthcare Improvement," Zeev Neuwirth podcast, November 5, 2017, http://shoutengine.com/CreatingaNewHealthcare/the-third-era-of-medicine-with-dr-don-berwick-pr-46122.

59 "Counting what Counts - Predictive Analytics & Artificial Intelligence in Healthcare with Len D'Avolio," Zeev Neuwirth podcast, January 11, 2018, http://shoutengine.com/CreatingaNewHealthcare/counting-what-counts-predictive-analytics-arti-49385

60 "Leadership Principles," Amazon Jobs, https://www.amazon.jobs/en/principles.

61 "Reframing chronic disease management - with George McLendon PhD, Founder of SensorRX; and VP for Therapeutics Research & Development at Atrium Health," Zeev Neuwirth podcast, February 9, 2018,

http://shoutengine.com/CreatingaNewHealthcare/reframing-chronic-disease-management-with-george-51393.

62   "Digital Behavioral Medicine with Sean Duffy, Co-founder & CEO of Omada Health," Zeev Neuwirth podcast, November 7, 2017, http://shoutengine.com/CreatingaNewHealthcare/digital-behavioral-medicine-with-sean-duffy-co-fo-46189.

63   Ibid.

64   Kyra Bobinet, *Well Designed Life: 10 Lessons in Brain Science & Design Thinking for a Mindful, Healthy, & Purposeful Life* (engagedIN Press, 2015).

Chapter 8

65   Regina Herzlinger, *Market-Driven Health Care* (Basic Books, 1999).

66   Michael E. Porter and Elizabeth Olmsted Teisberg, *Redefining Health Care: Creating Value-Based Competition on Results* (Harvard Business Review Press, 2006).

Chapter 9

67   "Digital Health with Sami Inkinen, Founder & CEO of Virta Health," Zeev Neuwirth podcast, (December 3, 2017), http://shoutengine.com/CreatingaNewHealthcare/digital-health-with-sami-inkinen-founder-ceo-of-47559.

68   "Insights into Creating a Model Healthcare System - w/ Dr. Mark Briesacher, Chief Physician Executive & President, Intermountain Med Group," Zeev Neuwirth podcast, May 4, 2018, http://shoutengine.com/CreatingaNewHealthcare/episode-36-insights-into-creating-a-model-health-57794.

69   "Walmart's consumer oriented healthcare transformation with Marcus Osborne," Zeev Neuwirth podcast, October 25, 2018,

http://shoutengine.com/CreatingaNewHealthcare/episode-48-walmarts-consumer-oriented-healthca-68068.

70 "Redefining what it means to be a Health Insurer, with Dr. Harold Paz," Zeev Neuwirth podcast, Oct. 11 2018, http://shoutengine.com/CreatingaNewHealthcare/episode-47-redefining-what-it-means-to-be-a-hea-67331.

71 Elaine Pofeldt, "Understanding clinically integrated networks," *Medical Economics*, February 10, 2016, http://www.medicaleconomics.com/technology/understanding-clinically-integrated-networks.

72 Alex Kacik, "Q&A with Amazon's Chris Holt on testing a consumer-first model in healthcare," Modern Healthcare, July 21, 2018, https://www.modernhealthcare.com/article/20180721/NEWS/180719898.

73 Christian Terwiesch, David A. Asch, and Kevin G. Volpp,"Technology and Medicine: Reimagining Provider Visits as the New Tertiary Care," *Annals of Internal Medicine*, 167 no. 11 (Dec 5, 2017): 814–815, http://annals.org/aim/article-abstract/2659602/technology-medicine-reimagining-provider-visits-new-tertiary-care.

Chapter 10

74 Glen Tullman, *On Our Terms: Empowering the New Health Consumer* (Magnusson-Skor Publishing, 2018).

75 https://www.virtahealth.com/

76 "Digital Health with Sami Inkinen, Founder & CEO of Virta Health," Zeev Neuwirth podcast, December 3, 2017, http://shoutengine.com/CreatingaNewHealthcare/digital-health-with-sami-inkinen-founder-ceo-of-47559.

77 "Consumerism in Healthcare with Kevan Mabbutt," Zeev Neuwirth podcast September 12, 2018, http://shoutengine.com/CreatingaNewHealthcare/episode-45-consumerism-in-healthcare-with-kevan-ma-65683.

78 Mitesh S. Patel, David A. Asch, and Kevin G. Volpp, "Wearable Devices as Facilitators, Not Drivers, of Health Behavior Change," *Journal of the American Medical Association*, 313, no. 5, (2015): 459-460. doi:10.1001/jama.2014.14781 https://jamanetwork.com/journals/jama/article-abstract/2089651.

79 Tina Reed, "It's not just Amazon: Employers are turning 'activist' when it comes to healthcare, *FierceHealthcare*, Sept 4, 2018, https://www.fiercehealthcare.com/hospitals-health-systems/it-s-not-just-amazon-employers-are-turning-activist-when-it-comes-to.

80 "The State Of Value In U.S. Health Care," University of Utah Health Survey, https://uofuhealth.utah.edu/value/.

81 "2018 Employer Health Benefits Survey," KFF, Henry J Kaiser Family Foundation, Oct 03, 2018, https://www.kff.org/report-section/2018-employer-health-benefits-survey-summary-of-findings.

82 Jay Hancock, "Why HDHPs are falling out of favor," BenefitsPro, October 5, 2018, https://www.benefitspro.com/2018/10/05/why-hdhps-are-falling-out-of-favor/?slreturn=20190026172958.

83 "A New 'True North' - An Economist's Perspective on Healthcare Costs and Spending," Zeev Neuwirth podcast, July 31, 2018, http://shoutengine.com/CreatingaNewHealthcare/a-new-true-north-an-economists-perspective-on-62950.

84 "Part I: Building a Value-based Employee Health Program with David Contorno," Zeev Neuwirth podcast, Nov 8, 2018, http://shoutengine.com/CreatingaNewHealthcare/episode-49-part-i-building-a-value-based-emplo-68792.

85 "Mercer U.S. National Survey of Employer-Sponsored Health Plans, Mercer, November 28, 2018, https://www.mercer.com/our-thinking/national-survey-of-employer-sponsored-health-plans.html.

86   Anna Wilde Mathews, "GM Cuts Different Type of Health-Care Deal," *The Wall Street Journal*, August 6, 2018, https://www.wsj.com/articles/gm-cuts-different-type-of-health-care-deal-1533582121.

87   Ed Emerman, "Large U.S. Employers Eye Changes to Health Care Delivery System as Cost to Provide Health Benefits Nears $15,000 per Employee," National Business Group on Health, August 7, 2018, https://www.businessgrouphealth.org/news/nbgh-news/press-releases/press-release-details/?ID=348.

88   "Best Practices in Health Care Employer Survey Report," Willis Towers Watson, January 31, 2018, https://www.willistowerswatson.com/en-US/insights/2018/01/2017-best-practices-in-health-care-employer-survey.

89   Reed Abelson, "The Last Company You Would Expect Is Reinventing Health Benefits (Frustrated with insurers, some large companies — including a certain cable behemoth — are shedding long-held practices and adopting a do-it-yourself approach.), *New York Times*, Aug 31 2018, https://www.nytimes.com/2018/08/31/health/comcast-health-insurance-employees.html.

90   "Best Practices in Health Care Employer Survey Report," Willis Towers Watson, January 31, 2018, https://www.willistowerswatson.com/en-US/insights/2018/01/2017-best-practices-in-health-care-employer-survey.

91   "HLTH (The Future of Healthcare); Generation Session, presentation by Lisa Woods and Marcus Osborne, Walmart," YouTube Video, posted June 4, 2018, https://www.youtube.com/watch?v=n87g_mb_kukhttps://hlth2018.com/speakers/lisa-woods/.

92   Elizabeth Zimmermann, "Mayo Clinic researchers demonstrate value of second opinions," *Mayo Clinic News Network*, August 4, 2017, https://newsnetwork.mayoclinic.org/discussion/mayo-clinic-researchers-demonstrate-value-of-second-opinions.

93　"Mercer U.S. National Survey of Employer-Sponsored Health Plans, Mercer, November 28, 2018, https://www.mercer.com/our-thinking/national-survey-of-employer-sponsored-health-plans.html.

94　Tina Reed, "It's not just Amazon: Employers are turning 'activist' when it comes to healthcare, FierceHealthcare, Sept 4, 2018, https://www.fiercehealthcare.com/hospitals-health-systems/it-s-not-just-amazon-employers-are-turning-activist-when-it-comes-to.

95　"The Cost of Employer-based Healthcare, with Dave Chase, co-founder and CEO of Health Rosetta," Zeev Neuwirth podcast, February 23, 2018, http://shoutengine.com/CreatingaNewHealthcare/the-cost-of-employer-based-healthcare-with-dave-c-53532.

96　"What is the Health Rosetta? The blueprint for high-performance health benefits," https://healthrosetta.org/health-rosetta/#basics.

97　Dave Chase and Tom Emerick, *CEO's Guide to Restoring the American Dream: How to deliver world class healthcare to your employees at half the cost* (Health Rosetta Media, 2017).

Chapter 11

98　Alex M. Azar II, "The Root of the Problem: America's Social Determinants of Health," *Hatch Foundation for Civility and Solutions*, November 14, 2018, https://www.hhs.gov/about/leadership/secretary/speeches/2018-speeches/the-root-of-the-problem-americas-social-determinants-of-health.html.

99　Steven A. Schroeder, "We Can Do Better - Improving the Health of the American People," *New England Journal of Medicine* 357 (September 20, 2007): 1221-1228, https://www.nejm.org/doi/full/10.1056/NEJMsa073350.

100　Richard Cooper, *Poverty and the Myths of Healthcare Reform* (Baltimore: Johns Hopkins University Press, 2016).

101 Raj Chetty et al., "The Association Between Income and Life Expectancy in the United States, 2001-2014," *Journal of the American Medical Association* 315, no. 16 (April 2016): 1750-1766, https://doi.org/10.1001/jama.2016.4226.

102 Laura Dwyer-Lindgren et al., "Inequalities in Life Expectancy Among US Counties, 1980 to 2014: Temporal Trends and Key Drivers," *Journal of the American Medical Association, Internal Medicine* 177, no. 7, (July 1, 2017): 1003-1011.

103 Richard Luscombe, "Life expectancy gap between rich and poor US regions is 'more than 20 years'," *The Guardian,* May 8, 2017, https://www.theguardian.com/inequality/2017/may/08/life-expectancy-gap-rich-poor-us-regions-more-than-20-years.

104 Lisa Esposito, "The Countless Ways Poverty Affects People's Health," *U.S. News & World Report,* April 20, 2016, https://health.usnews.com/health-news/patient-advice/articles/2016-04-20/the-countless-ways-poverty-affects-peoples-health.

105 Steven A. Schroeder, "We Can Do Better - Improving the Health of the American People," New England Journal of Medicine, 357, (September 20, 2007): 1221-1228, https://www.nejm.org/doi/full/10.1056/NEJMsa073350.

106 "Dr. David T. Feinberg says fixing healthcare is 'the simplest thing we can do'," Oct 9, 2018; *FIXING HEALTHCARE PODCAST,* October 9, 2018, https://fixinghealthcarepodcast.com/2018/10/09/episode-3/.

107 "Estimates of Diabetes and Its Burden in the United States," *National Diabetes Statistics Report, 2017,* https://www.cdc.gov/diabetes/pdfs/data/statistics/national-diabetes-statistics-report.pdf.

108 Ibid.

109 "Dr. David T. Feinberg says fixing healthcare is 'the simplest thing we can do'," Oct 9, 2018; FIXING HEALTHCARE PODCAST, October 9, 2018, https://fixinghealthcarepodcast.com/2018/10/09/episode-3.

110 Andrea T. Feinberg et al., "How Geisinger Treats Diabetes by Giving Away Free, Healthy Food," *Harvard Business Review*, October 25, 2017, https://hbr.org/2017/10/how-geisinger-treats-diabetes-by-giving-away-free-healthy-food.

111 Andrea T. Feinberg et al., "Prescribing Food as a Specialty Drug," *NEJM Catalyst*, April 10, 2018, https://catalyst.nejm.org/prescribing-fresh-food-farmacy.

112 "How Geisinger Thinks About Strategy - an interview with Dominic Moffa, EVP & Chief Strategy Officer for Geisinger,Neuwirth podcast, April 19, 2018, http://shoutengine.com/CreatingaNewHealthcare/episode-34-how-geisinger-thinks-about-strategy-56812.

113 Andrea T. Feinberg et al., "Prescribing Food as a Specialty Drug," NEJM Catalyst, April 10, 2018, https://catalyst.nejm.org/prescribing-fresh-food-farmacy.

114 "Dr. David T. Feinberg says fixing healthcare is 'the simplest thing we can do'," Oct 9, 2018; FIXING HEALTHCARE PODCAST, October 9, 2018, https://fixinghealthcarepodcast.com/2018/10/09/episode-3.

115 Jena McGregor, "This former surgeon general says there's a 'loneliness epidemic' and work is partly to blame," *The Washington Post*, October 4, 2017, https://www.washingtonpost.com/news/on-leadership/wp/2017/10/04/this-former-surgeon-general-says-theres-a-loneliness-epidemic-and-work-is-partly-to-blame/?noredirect=on&utm_term=.c77009de1f5f.

116 Vivek Murthy, "Work And The Loneliness Epidemic." *Harvard Business Review, the Big Idea*, 2017, https://hbr.org/cover-story/2017/09/work-and-the-loneliness-epidemic.

117 Holly Hedegaard, Arialdi M. Miniño, and Margaret Warner, "Drug Overdose Deaths in the United States, 1999–2017," National Center for Health Statistics, 2018, https://www.cdc.gov/nchs/products/databriefs/db329.htm.

118 "Health United States, 2017 with Special Feature on Mortality," National Center for Health Statistics, 2017, https://www.cdc.gov/nchs/data/hus/hus17.pdf.

119 "Suicide rising across the US," Centers for Disease Control and Prevention, https://www.cdc.gov/vitalsigns/suicide.

120 Steve H. Woolf and Laudan Aron, "Failing health of the United States – The role of challenging life conditions and the policies behind them", BMJ, February 2018), 360:k496.

121 Springboard Healthy Scranton, *Geisinger*, https://www.springboardhealthy.org/#Home.

122 "A Novel Approach to Harness the Most Powerful Social Determinants of Health," (with Michellene Davis) Zeev Neuwirth podcast, May 31, 2018, http://shoutengine.com/CreatingaNewHealthcare/episode-39-a-novel-approach-to-harness-the-most-59377.

123 I first learned about this network from Thompson and another highly accomplished, values-based leader – Michellene Davis, the Executive Vice President and Chief Corporate Affairs Officer at Robert Wood Johnson Saint Barnabas, the largest healthcare system in New Jersey.

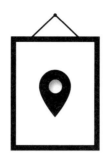

Chapter 1—"Houston We have a Problem"

Health United States, 2017 with Special Feature on Mortality https://www.cdc.gov/nchs/data/hus/hus17.pdf.

Papanicolas, L. R. Woskie, and A. K. Jha, "Health Care Spending in the United States and Other High-Income Countries," *Journal of the American Medical Association* 319, no. 10 (March 13, 2018):1024–39.

Drug Overdose Deaths in the United States 1999-2016 by Holly Hedegaard, M.D., Margaret Warner, Ph.D., and Arialdi M. Miniño, M.P.H.

https://www.cdc.gov/nchs/data/databriefs/db294.pdf

The CEO's Guide to Restoring: How to Deliver World Class Healthcare to Your Employees at Half the Cost by Dave Chase

Overtreated: Why Too Much Medicine Is Making Us Sicker and Poorer by Shannon Brownlee

Mistreated: Why We Think Were Getting Good Healthcare—and Why Were Usually Wrong by Robert Pearl

Ex-Acute: A Former Hospital CEO Tells All On What's Wrong With American Healthcare by Josh Luke

Crossing the Quality Chasm—Institute of Medicine

America's Bitter Pill: Money, Politics, Backroom Deals, and the Fight to Fix Our Healthcare System by Steven Brill

Catastrophic Care: Why Everything We Think We Know About Healthcare is Wrong by David Goldhill

An American Sickness: How Healthcare Became Big and How You Can Take it Back by Elisabeth Rosenthal

Demand Better: Revive Our Broken Healthcare System by Sanjaya Kumar, MD, MSc, MPH and David B. Nash, MD, MBA

Patients Come Second: Leading Change by Changing the Way You Lead by Paul Spiegelman and Britt Berett

Chapter 2—The Reframe Roadmap

Reengineering the Corporation: A Manifesto for Business Revolution by Michael Hammer and James Champy

Reengineering Healthcare: A Manifesto for Radically Rethinking Health Care Delivery by James Champy and Harry Greenspun MD

Digital Health with Sara Vaezy, Chief of Digital Strategy for Providence St. Joseph Health, Nov 16, 2017 (podcast)

http://shoutengine.com/CreatingaNewHealthcare/
digital-health-with-sara-vaezy-chief-of-digital-s-46704

Extreme Ownership: How U.S. Navy Seals Lead and Win by Jocko Willink and Leif Babin

The Essential Drucker by Peter Drucker

Better and Faster: The Proven Path to Unstoppable Ideas by Jeremy Gutsche

Man's Search for Meaning by Viktor Frankl

Where Good Ideas Come From by Johnson Steven

Seeing What Others Don't: The Remarkable Ways We Gain Insights by Gary Klein

The Black Swan by Nassim Nicholas Taleb

What Got You Here Won't Get You There by Marshall Goldsmith

Outliers: The Story of Success by Malcolm Gladwell

Chapter 3—The Marketing Mindset

The Innovator's Dilemma by Christensen

Redefining Health Care: Creating Value-Based Competition on Results by Michael E. Porter and Elizabeth Olmsted Teisberg

The Act of Creation, a Study of the Conscious and Unconscious in Science and Art by Arthur Koestler

The Structure of Scientific Revolutions: 50th Anniversary Edition by Thomas Kuhn

Chapter 4—Rebranding

Start With Why: How Great Leaders Inspire Everyone to Take Action by Simon Sinek

What do you call a 17-year old Ad Campaign? Priceless,

https://www.forbes.com/sites/avidan/2014/08/25/what-do-you-call-a-17-year-old-ad-campaign-priceless/#41f73c377142

The Hero's Journey: Joseph Campbell On His Life and Work by Joseph Campbell

The Hero with a Thousand Faces by Joseph Campbell

Building a Story Brand: Clarify Your Message So Customers Will Listen by Donald Miller

Brand Now: How to Stand Out in a Crowded, Distracted World by Nick Westergaard

It's Not What You Sell, It's What You Stand For: Why Every Extraordinary Business Is Driven by Purpose by Roy Spence

Brand Vs. Wild: Building Resilient Brands for Harsh Business Environments by Jonathan David Lewis

This Is Marketing: You Can't Be Seen Until You Learn to See by Seth Godin

The 22 Immutable Laws of Branding: How to Build a Product Or Service Into a World-Class Brand by Al Ries and Laura Ries

What Great Brands Do: The Seven Brand-Building Principles that Separate the Best from the Rest by Denise Lee Yohn

Chapter 5—Rebranding Primary Care

An online program for pediatric weight loss—with Joanna Strober, CEO of Kurbo, Sept 7, 2017, (podcast)

Chapter 6—Redesigning

Walmart's consumer oriented healthcare transformation with Marcus Osborne, Oct 25, 2018 (podcast)

http://shoutengine.com/CreatingaNewHealthcare/ episode-48-walmarts-consumer-oriented-healthca-68068

The Design of Everyday Things by Don Norman

The Power of Habit by Charles Duhigg

The Art of Innovation by Tom Kelley

The Ten Faces of Innovation by Tom Kelley

10 Rules for Strategic Innovators: From Idea to Execution by Vijay Govindarajan and Chris Trimble

The Startup Owner's Manual: The Step-By-Step Guide for Building a Great Company by Steve Blank and Bob Dorf

Change By Design: How Design Thinking Transforms Organizations and Inspires Innovation by Tim Brown

Chapter 7—Principles of Redesigning

Managing for Results by Peter Drucker

The Laws of Simplicity by John Maeda

Essentialism: The Disciplined Pursuit of Less by Greg McKeown

The One Thing: The Surprisingly Simple Truth Behind Extraordinary Results by Gary Keller and Jay Papasan

Predictably Irrational, Revised and Expanded Edition: The Hidden Forces That Shape Our Decisions by Dan Ariely

Thinking Fast and Slow by Daniel Kahneman

Nudge: Improving Decisions about Health, Wealth and Happiness by Richard H. Thaler and Cass R. Sustien

Willpower: Rediscovering the Greatest Human Strength by Roy F. Baumeister and John Tierney

The Wisdom of Crowds: Why the Many are Smarter than the Few and How Collective Wisdom Shapes Business, Economics, Societies, and Nations by James Surowiecki

Learned Optimism by Martin E. P. Seligman PhD

Hooked: How to Build Habit by Nir Eyal

Mitesh S. Patel, "Effect of a Game-Based Intervention Designed to Enhance Social Incentives to Increase Physical Activity Among Families The BE FIT Randomized Clinical Trial," *JAMA Intern Med* 177, no. 11 (Nov. 2017): 1586–1593, https://doi.org/10.1001/jamainternmed.2017.3458, https://jamanetwork.com/journals/jamainternalmedicine/fullarticle/2655242?resultClick=1.

Neel P. Chokshi et al., "Loss-Framed Financial Incentives and Personalized Goal-Setting to Increase Physical Activity Among Ischemic Heart Disease Patients Using Wearable Devices: The ACTIVE REWARD Randomized Trial," *Journal of the American Heart*

Association 7, no. 12 (June 2018), https://www.ahajournals.org/
doi/10.1161/JAHA.118.009173.

Chapter 8—Reorganizing

Market-Driven Healthcare by Regina Herzlinger

Consumers, Corporations and Public Health by John A. Quelch

Business Model Generation by Alexander Osterwalder and Yves
Pigneur

Antifragile: Things That Gain from Disorder by Nassim Nicholas Taleb

Zero to One: Notes on Startups, or How to Build the Future by Peter
Thiel with Blake Masters

Chapter 9—Reorganizing's Disruptive Potential

Antoine Gara, "Healthcare Stocks Plunge As Buffett, Bezos And Dimon
Team Up To Fight 'Tapeworm' Costs On Economy," *Forbes*, January
30, 2018, https://www.forbes.com/sites/antoinegara/2018/01/30/
healthcare-stocks-plunge-as-buffett-bezos-and-dimon-team-up-to-
fight-tapeworm-costs-on-economy/#1864ddf65319

Chapter 10—Game-Changing Trends

*Competitive Strategy: Techniques for Analyzing Industries and Competi-
tors* by Michael E. Porter

Diffusion of Innovation, 5th ed. by Everett M. Rogers

The Patient Will See You Now: The Future of Medicine Is in Your Hands by Eric Topol

The Digital Doctor: Hope, Hype, and Harm at the Dawn of Medicine's Computer Age by Robert M. Wachter

The Creative Destruction of Medicine by Eric Topol

Chapter 11- Social Determinants of Health

Poverty and The Myths of Healthcare Reform: Why Poverty and Income Inequality Are at the Core of America'sHigh Health Care Spending by Richard Cooper

Diagnosis: Poverty: A New Approach to Understanding and Treating an Epidemic by Marcella Wilson PhD

Evicted: Poverty and Profit in the American City by Matthew Desmond

ProvenCare: How to Deliver Value-Based Healthcare the Geisinger Way by Glenn D. Steeler Jr. MD and David T. Feinberg, MD

The Illness Narratives by Arthur Kleinman MD

Epilogue

Heretics to Heroes: A Memoir on Modern Leadership by Dial Cort

Lead True—Live Your Values, Build Your People, Inspire Your Community by Jeff Thompson MD

Value Based Leadership with Dr. Jeff Thompson, Dec 5, 2018 (podcast), http://shoutengine.com/CreatingaNewHealthcare/episode-52-value-based-leadership-with-dr-jeff-70128

Lessons on Healthcare Media & Leadership—with Scott Becker, founder & publisher of the Becker's Healthcare & Becker's Hospital Review, April 10, 2018 (podcast), http://shoutengine.com/CreatingaNewHealthcare/episode-33-lessons-on-healthcare-media-leader-56190

How Will You Measure Your Life? by Clayton M. Christensen

The Obstacle Is the Way: The Timeless Art of Turning Trials into Triumph by Ryan Holiday

Leadership Without Easy Answers by Ronald A. Heifetz

Dare to Lead, Daring Greatly, and *Rising Strong at Work* by Brene Brown

Originals: How Non-Conformists Move the World by Adam Grant

Leading Change by John P. Kotter

Influencer: The New Science of Leading Change by Joseph Grenny, Kerry Patterson, David Maxfield, Ron McMillan, and Al Switzler

Multipliers: How the Best Leaders Make Everyone Smarter by Liz Wiseman with Greg McKeown